Nursing Calculations

Ninth edition

J. D. Gatford
Mathematics Tutor, Melbourne, Australia

N. M. Phillips
DipAppSc(Nsg) BN GDipAdvNsg(Educ) MNS PhD
Associate Professor, Director of Undergraduate Studies, School of
Nursing and Midwifery, Deakin University, Victoria, Australia

ELSEVIER

Edinburgh   London   New York   Oxford   Philadelphia   St Louis   Sydney   Toronto   2016

ELSEVIER

First edition 1982   Fifth edition 1998
Second edition 1987   Sixth edition 2002
Third edition 1990   Seventh edition 2006
Fourth edition 1994   Eighth edition 2011 (Reprinted twice)

ISBN 978-0-7020-6231-5

Notices

 ELSEVIER your source for books, journals and multimedia in the health sciences

www.elsevierhealth.com

  Working together to grow libraries in developing countries

www.elsevier.com • www.bookaid.org

The publisher's policy is to use **paper manufactured from sustainable forests**

Printed in China

Nursing

ns

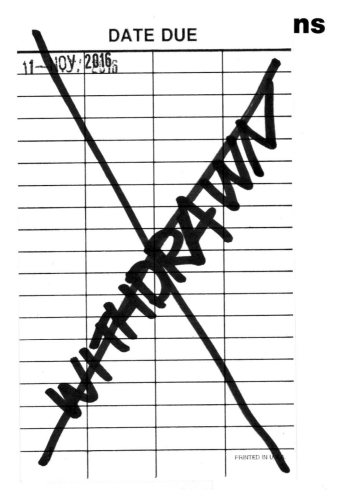

For Elsevier

Content Strategist: Alison Taylor
Content Development Specialist: Veronika Watkins
Project Manager: Joanna Souch
Designer: Christian Bilbow
Illustration Manager: Karen Giacomucci

Contents

Preface to the Ninth Edition

In this new edition, all questions have been reviewed and updated where necessary to reflect current practice. Some additional questions have been included and prescriptions using a medication chart have been incorporated into questions that involve medication labels.

A 24-hour time chart has been added to Chapter 1. Additional worked examples have been included to facilitate understanding of the use of 24-hour time. An additional revision exercise has been included in Chapter 6 to provide further practice of all calculations covered in the book.

Please note that the aim of *Nursing Calculations* is to teach relevant skills in *arithmetic*; the book is *not* meant to be used as a pharmacology reference.

John Gatford and Nicole Phillips
Melbourne 2016

Preface to the First Edition

This book was written at the request of nurse educators and with considerable help from them. It deals with elements of the arithmetic of nursing, especially the arithmetic of basic pharmacology.

The book begins with a diagnostic test which is carefully related to a set of review exercises in basic arithmetic. Answers to the test are supplied at the back of the book, and are keyed to the corresponding review exercises.

Students should work through those exercises which correspond to errors in the diagnostic test. The other exercises may also, of course, be worked through to improve speed and accuracy.

Throughout the other chapters of the book there are adequate, well-graded exercises and problems. Each chapter includes several worked examples. Answers are given to all questions.

Suggestions and comments from nurse educators and students on the scope and content of this book would be welcomed. The hope is that its relevance to nursing needs will be maintained in subsequent editions.

J.D.G.
Melbourne 1982

Acknowledgements

The authors would like to thank those nurse educators, nurses and pharmacists who provided advice and suggestions during the preparation of this ninth edition. Special thanks to Rebecca Thornton, lecturer in the School of Nursing and Midwifery at Deakin University, for her paediatric advice.

The authors wish also to thank Alison Taylor, Senior Commissioning Editor for Nursing and Midwifery at Elsevier Ltd, who recommended a ninth edition; Veronika Watkins, Content Development Specialist, who managed the project; Meg Bayley, Diabetic Educator; Gavin Hawkins, for the syringe graphics; and Matthew Gatford for checking the answers to Chapter 1.

We are grateful to the Sanofi–Aventis Group and to GlaxoSmithKline Australia Pty Ltd for permission to reproduce medication labels for inclusion in this book. Thank you to the Australian Commission on Safety and Quality in Health Care for granting permission to use the National Inpatient Medication Chart – Acute (2012).

John Gatford wishes to thank his wife, Elaine, for her continuing support and patience during this ongoing project.

Thanks also, from Nicole Phillips, to Theo, Curtis, and Taylor.

Useful abbreviations

BSA	body surface area
cm	centimetre(s)
d.p.	decimal place(s)
g	gram(s)
hr(s)	hour(s)
hrly	hourly
IM	intramuscular
IV	intravenous
kg	kilogram(s)
kJ	kilojoule(s)
L	litre(s)
m^2	square metre(s)
mg	milligram(s)
mg/m^2	milligram(s) per square metre
mg/mL	milligrams per millilitre
mg/kg/day	milligrams per kilogram per day
min	minute(s)
mL	millilitre(s)
mL/hr	millilitres per hour
PCA	patient controlled analgesia
PO	orally
stat	immediately
subcut	subcutaneous
WFI	water-for-injection
%	percentage

Note: *Do not use an abbreviation for micrograms.*

Formulae used in this book

$$\text{Volume required (VR)} = \frac{\text{Strength required (SR)}}{\text{Stock strength (SS)}} \times \begin{bmatrix} \text{Volume of} \\ \text{stock solution (VS)} \end{bmatrix}$$

$$\text{Volume (mL)} = \text{Rate (mL/hr)} \times \text{Time (hr)}$$

$$\text{Time (hr)} = \frac{\text{Volume (mL)}}{\text{Rate (mL/hr)}}$$

$$\text{Rate (mL/hr)} = \frac{\text{Volume (mL)}}{\text{Time (hr)}}$$

$$\text{Rate (mL/hr)} = \frac{\text{Volume (mL)} \times 60}{\text{Time (min)}}$$

$$\text{Rate (drops/min)} = \frac{\text{Volume (mL)} \times \text{Drop factor (drops/mL)}}{\text{Time (minutes)}}$$

$$\text{Rate (drops/min)} = \frac{\text{Volume (mL)} \times \text{Drop factor (drops/mL)}}{\text{Time (hours)} \times 60}$$

$$\text{Running time (hours)} = \frac{\text{Volume (mL)}}{\text{Rate (mL/hr)}}$$

$$\text{Concentration of stock (mg/mL)} = \frac{\text{Stock strength (mg)}}{\text{Volume of stock solution (mL)}}$$

$$\text{Dosage (mg)} = \text{Volume (mL)} \times \text{Concentration of stock (mg/mL)}$$

$$\text{Hourly dosage (mg/hr)} = \text{Rate (mL/hr)} \times \text{Concentration of stock (mg/mL)}$$

$$\text{Rate (mL/hr)} = \frac{\text{Hourly dosage (mg/hr)}}{\text{Concentration of stock (mg/mL)}}$$

$$\text{Weight of dextrose (g)} = \text{Volume of infusion (mL)} \times \text{strength of solution (g/100 mL)}$$

$$\text{Dose required (mg)} = \text{Body surface area (m}^2\text{)} \times \text{Recommended dosage (mg/m}^2\text{)}$$

A review of relevant calculations

In this chapter, a list of mathematical terms is followed by a diagnostic test. This test is designed to pinpoint those areas of your arithmetic that need revising before you start nursing calculations. The test identifies what you already understand and what you need to review.

You should attempt all questions in the diagnostic test.

Answers are provided in Chapter 7. According to the incorrect answers in your diagnostic test, you will be directed to particular review exercises.

For example, if you make an error in answering either test question 1 or test question 2, then you will be directed to do Review exercise 1A. Or, if your answer to test question 3 or 4 is wrong, you should do Review exercise 1B. You will not need to review any skills that the diagnostic test shows you already know.

Remember that this test is designed to help you.

Refer to prelim page ix for explanations of abbreviations.

CHAPTER CONTENTS

SHORT LIST OF MATHEMATICAL TERMS

WHOLE NUMBERS

Whole number: A number without fractions.

e.g. 5, 17, 438, 10 592

FRACTIONS

e.g. $\frac{3}{8}$ $\frac{17}{5}$ $\frac{1}{6}$ $\frac{9}{4000}$

Numerator: The top number in a fraction.

e.g. In the fraction $\frac{3}{8}$ the numerator is 3.

Denominator: The bottom number in a fraction.

e.g. In the fraction $\frac{3}{8}$ the denominator is 8.

PROPER AND IMPROPER FRACTIONS

Proper fraction: A fraction in which the numerator is smaller than the denominator.

e.g. $\frac{1}{4}$ $\frac{5}{8}$ $\frac{11}{100}$

Improper fraction: A fraction in which the numerator is larger than the denominator.

e.g. $\frac{5}{3}$ $\frac{32}{7}$ $\frac{100}{9}$

An improper fraction can be converted to a mixed number.

e.g. $\frac{5}{3} = 1\frac{2}{3}$ $\frac{32}{7} = 4\frac{4}{7}$ $\frac{100}{9} = 11\frac{1}{9}$

Mixed number: Partly a whole number, partly a fraction.

e.g. $1\frac{5}{8}$ $4\frac{1}{2}$ $10\frac{4}{5}$

A mixed number can be converted to an improper fraction.

e.g. $1\frac{5}{8} = \frac{13}{8}$ $4\frac{1}{2} = \frac{9}{2}$ $10\frac{4}{5} = \frac{54}{5}$

DECIMALS

Decimal: A number that includes a decimal point.

e.g. 6.35, 0.748, 0.002, 236.5

Decimal places: Numbers to the right of the decimal point.

e.g. 6.35 has 2 decimal places.
   0.748 has 3 decimal places.
   0.002 has 3 decimal places.
   236.5 has 1 decimal place.

Place value

To the right of the decimal point are tenths, hundredths, thousandths, etc.

e.g. In the number 0.962, there are 9 tenths, 6 hundredths and 2 thousandths.

PERCENTAGES

Percentage: Number of parts per hundred parts.

e.g. 14% means 14 parts per 100 parts.
   2.5% means 2.5 parts per 100 parts.

A percentage may be less than 1%.

e.g. 0.3% = 0.3 parts per 100 = 3 parts per 1000
   0.04% = 0.04 parts per 100 = 4 parts per 10000

OTHER TERMS

Divisor: The number by which you are dividing.

e.g. In the division 495 ÷ 15, the divisor is 15.

Factors

When a number is divided by one of its factors, the answer is a whole number (i.e. there is no remainder).

e.g.   The factors of 12 are 1, 2, 3, 4, 6 and 12.
The factors of 20 are 1, 2, 4, 5, 10 and 20.
The number 1 is a factor of every number.

Common factors

Two different numbers may have common factors – factors that are common to both numbers.

e.g. 1, 2 and 4 are the common factors of 12 and 20.

Simplify: Write as simply as possible.

Calculate the value of: The answer will be a number.

DIAGNOSTIC TEST

1   Multiply
    a 83×10 **b** 83×100 **c** 83×1000

2   Multiply
    a 0.0258×10 **b** 0.0258×100 **c** 0.0258×1000

3   Divide. Write answers as decimals.
    a $3.78 \div 10$ **b** $3.78 \div 100$ **c** $3.78 \div 1000$

4   Divide. Write answers as decimals.
    a $\dfrac{569}{10}$ **b** $\dfrac{569}{100}$ **c** $\dfrac{569}{1000}$

5   Complete
    a 1 kilogram = ………………….. grams

    b 1 gram = ………………….. milligrams

    c 1 milligram = ………………….. micrograms

    d 1 litre = ………………….. millilitres

Write answers to 6, 7, 8 and 9 in decimal form.

6   **a** Change 0.83 kilograms to grams.

    b Change 6400 g to kg.

7   **a** Change 0.78 grams to milligrams.

    b Change 34 milligrams to grams.

8   **a** Change 0.086 milligrams to micrograms.

    b Change 294 micrograms to milligrams.

9   **a** Change 2.4 litres to millilitres.

    b Change 965 millilitres to litres.

10 **a** Change 0.07 L to mL.

    b Change 0.007 L to mL.

    c Which is larger: 0.07 L or 0.007 L?

Check your answers on p 143

11   a Convert 0.045 g to mg.

     b Convert 0.45 g to mg.

     c Which is heavier: 0.045 g or 0.45 g?

12 Multiply

     a 9×3 b 0.9×3

     c 0.9×0.3 d 0.09×0.03

13 Multiply

     a 78×6 b 7.8×0.6

     c 0.78×6 d 7.8×0.06

14 Which of the numbers 2, 3, 4, 5, 6, 10, 12 are **factors** of 48?

15 Which of the numbers 2, 3, 5, 6, 7, 9, 11 are **factors** of 126?

16 Simplify ('cancel down')

     a $\dfrac{16}{24}$ b $\dfrac{56}{72}$

17 Simplify

     a $\dfrac{45}{600}$ b $\dfrac{175}{400}$

18 Simplify

     a $\dfrac{40}{50}$ b $\dfrac{60}{90}$ c $\dfrac{90}{150}$

19 Simplify

     a $\dfrac{350}{500}$ b $\dfrac{1200}{1500}$ c $\dfrac{1600}{4000}$

20 Simplify ('cancel down'). Leave answers as improper fractions.

     a $\dfrac{65}{20}$ b $\dfrac{275}{50}$ c $\dfrac{500}{80}$

Check your answers on p 143

Nursing Calculations

21 Simplify ('cancel down'). Leave answers as improper fractions.

a $\dfrac{700}{120}$ b $\dfrac{400}{125}$ c $\dfrac{600}{250}$

22 Simplify. Leave answers as improper fractions, where these occur.

a $\dfrac{0.6}{0.9}$ b $\dfrac{0.45}{0.5}$

c $\dfrac{200}{4.5}$ d $\dfrac{0.09}{0.05}$

23 Round off each number correct to one decimal place.

a 0.68   b 1.82   c 0.35

24 Write each number correct to two decimal places.

a 0.374   b 2.625   c 0.516

25 Change to exact decimal equivalents.

a $\dfrac{5}{8}$ b $\dfrac{9}{20}$

c $\dfrac{17}{25}$ d $\dfrac{31}{40}$

26 Change to decimals correct to one decimal place.

a $\dfrac{1}{6}$ b $\dfrac{3}{7}$ c $\dfrac{7}{9}$

27 Change to decimals correct to two decimal places.

a $\dfrac{5}{7}$ b $\dfrac{5}{9}$

28 Divide. Calculate the value of each fraction to the nearest whole number.

a $\dfrac{95}{3}$ b $\dfrac{225}{4}$

Check your answers on pp 143–144

29 Divide. Calculate the value of each fraction correct to one decimal place.

a $\dfrac{55}{6}$ b $\dfrac{65}{9}$

30 Change to mixed numbers.

a $\dfrac{17}{2}$ b $\dfrac{67}{3}$ c $\dfrac{113}{5}$

31 Change to improper fractions.

a $2\tfrac{3}{4}$ b $12\tfrac{5}{6}$ c $28\tfrac{2}{5}$

32 Multiply. Simplify where possible.

a $\dfrac{2}{3}\times\dfrac{5}{6}$ b $\dfrac{5}{8}\times\dfrac{12}{7}$ c $\dfrac{9}{10}\times\dfrac{4}{9}$

33 Multiply. Simplify where possible. Write each answer as a fraction, a mixed number, or a whole number.

a $\dfrac{5}{4}\times 3$ b $\dfrac{5}{8}\times 4$

34 Multiply. Give each answer as a decimal number.

a $\dfrac{11}{20}\times 4$ b $\dfrac{30}{50}\times 2$

35 Convert to 24-hour time.

a 10:30 am   b 9:15 pm

36 Convert to am/pm time.

a 0730 hours   b 1850 hours

37 What is the time 10 hours after 2145 hours on a Saturday?

Check your answers on p 144

MULTIPLICATION BY 10, 100 AND 1000

To multiply by 10, move the decimal point 1 place to the right.

To multiply by 100, move the decimal point 2 places to the right.

To multiply by 1000, move the decimal point 3 places to the right.

Example

a	**0.36 × 10**	a	$0.36 \times 10 = 3.6$	$= 3.6$
b	**0.36 × 100**	b	$0.36 \times 100 = 36.$	$= 36$
c	**0.36 × 1000**	c	$0.36 \times 1000 = 360.$	$= 360$

Notes:

- Use zeros to make up places, where necessary.
- If the answer is a whole number, the decimal point may be omitted.

Memorise

To multiply by	Move the decimal point
10	1 place right
100	2 places right
1000	3 places right

Review exercise 1A *Multiply*

1 0.68×10
   0.68×100
   0.68×1000

2 0.975×10
   0.975×100
   0.975×1000

3 3.7×10
   3.7×100
   3.7×1000

4 5.62×10
   5.62×100
   5.62×1000

5 77×10
   77×100
   77×1000

6 825×10
   825×100
   825×1000

7 0.2×10
   0.2×100
   0.2×1000

8 0.046×10
   0.046×100
   0.046×1000

9 0.0147×10
   0.0147×100
   0.0147×1000

10 0.006×10
    0.006×100
    0.006×1000

11 3.76×10
    3.76×100
    3.76×1000

12 0.639×10
    0.639×100
    0.639×1000

13 0.075×10
    0.075×100
    0.075×1000

14 0.08×10
    0.08×10
    0.08×1000

15 0.003×10
    0.003×100
    0.003×1000

16 0.0505×10
    0.0505×100
    0.0505×1000

Check your answers on p 144

DIVISION BY 10, 100 AND 1000

To divide by 10, move the decimal point 1 place to the left.

To divide by 100, move the decimal point 2 places to the left.

To divide by 1000, move the decimal point 3 places to the left.

Example A

a 37.8 ÷ 10

b 37.8 ÷ 100

c 37.8 ÷ 1000

a $37.8 \div 10 = 3.78 = 3.78$

b $37.8 \div 100 = 0.378 = 0.378$

c $37.8 \div 1000 = 0.0378 = 0.0378$

Notes:

• Use zeros to make up places, where necessary.
• For numbers less than one, write a zero before the decimal point.

Example B

A division may be written as a fraction.

a $\dfrac{0.984}{10}$

b $\dfrac{0.984}{100}$

c $\dfrac{0.984}{1000}$

a $\dfrac{0.984}{10} = 0.0984$

b $\dfrac{0.984}{100} = 0.00984$

c $\dfrac{0.984}{1000} = 0.000984$

Memorise

To divide by	Move the decimal point
10	1 place left
100	2 places left
1000	3 places left

Review exercise 1B *Divide. Write answers as decimals.*

1 98.4 ÷ 10
   98.4 ÷ 100
   98.4 ÷ 1000

2 5.91 ÷ 10
   5.91 ÷ 100
   5.91 ÷ 1000

3 2.6 ÷ 10
   2.6 ÷ 100
   2.6 ÷ 1000

4 307 ÷ 10
   307 ÷ 100
   307 ÷ 1000

5 82 ÷ 10
   82 ÷ 100
   82 ÷ 1000

6 7 ÷ 10
   7 ÷ 100
   7 ÷ 1000

7 3 ÷ 10
   3 ÷ 100
   3 ÷ 1000

8 7.5 ÷ 10
   7.5 ÷ 100
   7.5 ÷ 1000

9 $\dfrac{68}{10}$

   $\dfrac{68}{100}$

   $\dfrac{68}{1000}$

10 $\dfrac{2.29}{10}$

   $\dfrac{2.29}{100}$

   $\dfrac{2.29}{1000}$

11 $\dfrac{51.4}{10}$

   $\dfrac{51.4}{100}$

   $\dfrac{51.4}{1000}$

12 $\dfrac{916}{10}$

   $\dfrac{916}{100}$

   $\dfrac{916}{1000}$

13 $\dfrac{67.2}{10}$

   $\dfrac{67.2}{100}$

   $\dfrac{67.2}{1000}$

14 $\dfrac{387}{10}$

   $\dfrac{387}{100}$

   $\dfrac{387}{1000}$

15 $\dfrac{8.94}{10}$

   $\dfrac{8.94}{100}$

   $\dfrac{8.94}{1000}$

16 $\dfrac{0.707}{10}$

   $\dfrac{0.707}{100}$

   $\dfrac{0.707}{1000}$

Check your answers on p 145

CONVERTING UNITS

Memorise

> 1 kilogram (kg) = 1000 grams (g)
> 1 gram (g) = 1000 milligrams (mg)
> 1 milligram (mg) = 1000 micrograms*
> 1 litre (L) = 1000 millilitres (mL)

*__Note:__ Always write micrograms in full.

Example A *Kilograms to grams*

Change 0.6 kg to grams.

$$0.6\,\text{kg} = 0.6 \times 1000\,\text{g}$$
$$= 600\,\text{g}$$

Example B *Grams to kilograms*

Change 375 g to kilograms.

$$375\,\text{g} = 375 \div 1000\,\text{kg}$$
$$= 0.375\,\text{kg}$$

Example C *Grams to milligrams*

Change 0.67 g to milligrams.

$$0.67\,\text{g} = 0.67 \times 1000\,\text{mg}$$
$$= 670\,\text{mg}$$

Example D *Milligrams to grams*

Change 23 mg to grams.

$$23\,\text{mg} = 23 \div 1000\,\text{g}$$
$$= 0.023\,\text{g}$$

Example E *Milligrams to micrograms*

Change 0.075 mg to micrograms.

$$0.075\,\text{mg} = 0.075 \times 1000\,\text{micrograms}$$
$$= 75\,\text{micrograms}$$

Example F *Micrograms to milligrams*

Change 185 micrograms to milligrams.

$$185\,\text{micrograms} = 185 \div 1000\,\text{mg}$$
$$= 0.185\,\text{mg}$$

Example G *Litres to millilitres*

Change 1.3 L to millilitres.

$$1.3\,\text{L} = 1.3 \times 1000\,\text{mL}$$
$$= 1300\,\text{mL}$$

Example H *Millilitres to litres*

Change 850 mL to litres.

$$850\,\text{mL} = 850 \div 1000\,\text{L}$$
$$= 0.85\,\text{L}$$

Review exercise 1C *Change (convert). Write all answers in decimal form.*

Change to grams.

1	5 kg	2	2.4 kg	3	0.75 kg	4	1.625 kg

Change to kilograms.

5	7000 g	6	935 g	7	85 g	8	3 g

Change to milligrams.

9	4 g	10	8.7 g	11	0.69 g	12	0.02 g
13	0.035 g	14	0.006 g	15	0.655 g	16	4.28 g

Change to grams.

17	6000 mg	18	7250 mg	19	865 mg	20	95 mg
21	70 mg	22	2 mg	23	5 mg	24	125 mg

Change to micrograms.

25	0.195 mg	26	0.6 mg	27	0.75 mg	28	0.075 mg
29	0.08 mg	30	0.001 mg	31	0.625 mg	32	0.098 mg

Change to milligrams.

33	825 micrograms	34	750 micrograms
35	65 micrograms	36	95 micrograms
37	10 micrograms	38	5 micrograms
39	200 micrograms	40	30 micrograms

Change to millilitres.

41	2 L	42	30 L	43	$1\frac{1}{2}$ L	44	$4\frac{1}{2}$ L
45	1.6 L	46	2.24 L	47	0.8 L	48	0.75 L

Change to litres.

49	4000 mL	50	10 000 mL	51	625 mL	52	350 mL
53	95 mL	54	60 mL	55	5 mL	56	2 mL

Check your answers on p 145

Nursing Calculations

COMPARING MEASUREMENTS

Example A

a   Change 0.4 L to mL.
b   Change 0.04 L to mL.
c   Which is larger: 0.4 L or 0.04 L?

1 L = 1000 mL

a $0.4 \text{ L} = 0.4 \times 1000 \text{ mL} = 400 \text{ mL}$
b $0.04 \text{ L} = 0.04 \times 1000 \text{ mL} = 40 \text{ mL}$
c   0.4 L is larger than 0.04 L

Example B

a   Convert 4.3 kg to grams.
b   Convert 4.03 kg to grams.
c   Which is heavier: 4.3 kg or 4.03 kg?

1 kg = 1000 g

a $4.3 \text{ kg} = 4.3 \times 1000 \text{ g} = 4300 \text{ g}$
b $4.03 \text{ kg} = 4.03 \times 1000 \text{ g} = 4030 \text{ g}$
c   4.3 kg is heavier than 4.03 kg

Review exercise 1D *Change and compare*

Change each given measurement to the smaller unit required. Then for part c choose the larger of the two given measurements.

Change each measurement to millilitres (mL); then choose the larger volume (c).

1	a 0.1 L	b 0.01 L	c
2	a 0.003 L	b 0.3 L	c
3	a 0.05 L	b 0.005 L	c
4	a 0.047 L	b 0.47 L	c

Convert each measurement to milligrams (mg); then choose the larger weight (c).

5	a 0.4 g	b 0.004 g	c
6	a 0.06 g	b 0.6 g	c
7	a 0.07 g	b 0.007 g	c
8	a 0.63 g	b 0.063 g	c

Rewrite each measurement in micrograms; then choose the bigger weight (c).

9	a 0.002 mg	b 0.02 mg	c
10	a 0.9 mg	b 0.09 mg	c
11	a 0.001 mg	b 0.1 mg	c
12	a 0.58 mg	b 0.058 mg	c

Change each measurement to grams (g); then choose the heavier weight (c).

13	a 1.5 kg	b 1.05 kg	c
14	a 2.08 kg	b 2.8 kg	c
15	a 0.95 kg	b 0.095 kg	c
16	a 3.35 kg	b 3.5 kg	c

Check your answers on p 146

MULTIPLICATION OF DECIMALS

Note: d.p. stands for decimal place(s).

Example A   ### Example B

a 8×4 a 67×4
b 0.8×4 b 6.7×0.4
c 0.8×0.4 c 0.67×4
d 0.08×0.04 d 6.7×0.04

a $8 \times 4 = 32$ a $67 \times 4 = 268$
b $0.8 \times 4 = 3.2$ b $6.7 \times 0.4 = 2.68$

    1 d.p. + 0 d.p. $\Rightarrow$ 1 d.p.   1 d.p. + 1 d.p. $\Rightarrow$ 2 d.p.

c $0.8 \times 0.4 = 0.32$ c $0.67 \times 4 = 2.68$

    1 d.p. + 1 d.p. $\Rightarrow$ 2 d.p.   2 d.p. + 0 d.p. $\Rightarrow$ 2 d.p.

d $0.08 \times 0.04 = 0.0032$ d $6.7 \times 0.04 = 0.268$

    2 d.p. + 2 d.p. $\Rightarrow$ 4 d.p.   1 d.p. + 2 d.p. $\Rightarrow$ 3 d.p.

Example C

a 16×12 a $16 \times 12 = 192$
b 1.6×1.2 b $1.6 \times 1.2 = 1.92$ (2 d.p.)
c 0.16×0.12 c $0.16 \times 0.12 = 0.0192$ (4 d.p.)
d 0.016×1.2 d $0.016 \times 1.2 = 0.0192$ (4 d.p.)

Review exercise 1E *Multiply*

1 9×5
   0.9×5
   0.9×0.5
   9×0.05

2 2×7
   0.2×0.7
   0.2×0.07
   0.02×0.07

3 3×4
   3×0.04
   0.3×0.4
   0.03×0.04

4 6×6
   0.6×0.6
   0.06×0.06
   0.6×0.006

5 7×8
   0.7×8
   0.7×0.8
   0.07×0.08

6 17×6
   1.7×6
   0.17×6
   0.17×0.6

7 19×8
   19×0.8
   0.19×0.8
   1.9×0.08

8 23×2
   2.3×0.2
   2.3×0.02
   2.3×0.002

9 29×5
   0.29×5
   2.9×0.5
   29×0.05

10 31×3
   3.1×0.3
   0.31×0.03
   31×0.003

11 37×9
   3.7×9
   3.7×0.09
   0.37×0.09

12 41×7
   0.41×0.7
   0.41×0.07
   4.1×0.7

13 48×4
   0.48×0.04
   48×0.004
   0.048×0.4

14 56×11
   5.6×1.1
   0.56×0.11
   56×0.011

15 64×12
   6.4×0.12
   0.64×0.12
   0.064×1.2

Check your answers on p 146

FACTORS

Many calculations involve the simplifying (or 'cancelling down') of fractions.

This requires a knowledge of *factors*. When a number is divided by one of its factors, the answer is a whole number (i.e. there is no remainder).

The symbol $\therefore$ means 'therefore'.

Example

Which of the numbers 2, 3, 5, 7, 11 are factors of 154?

$\overline{2)\,154}$

77 [no remainder]

$\therefore$ 2 *is* a factor of 154

$\overline{3)\,154}$

51 + 1 remainder

$\therefore$ 3 *is not* a factor of 154

$\overline{5)\,154}$

30 + 4 remainder

$\therefore$ 5 *is not* a factor of 154

$\overline{7)\,154}$

22 [no remainder]

$\therefore$ 7 *is* a factor of 154

$\overline{11)\,154}$

14 [no remainder]

$\therefore$ 11 *is* a factor of 154

2, 7 and 11 are factors of 154.

Notes:

- These are not the *only* factors of 154.
- The numbers can, of course, be checked mentally!

Review exercise 1F *Which of the numbers in column B are factors of the opposite number in column A?*

	A	B
1	20	2, 3, 4, 5, 7, 8
2	36	3, 4, 5, 10, 12, 16
3	45	3, 5, 7, 11, 12, 15
4	56	2, 5, 8, 11, 14, 16
5	60	3, 4, 8, 12, 15, 20
6	72	3, 4, 6, 12, 15, 18
7	75	3, 5, 7, 11, 15, 25
8	85	3, 5, 9, 11, 15, 17
9	96	3, 8, 12, 14, 16, 24
10	100	3, 5, 8, 20, 25, 40
11	108	4, 7, 9, 12, 16, 18
12	120	3, 5, 9, 12, 15, 16
13	135	3, 5, 7, 9, 11, 15
14	144	4, 8, 12, 16, 18, 24
15	150	4, 5, 9, 12, 15, 25
16	165	3, 5, 7, 9, 11, 15
17	175	3, 5, 7, 9, 11, 15
18	180	4, 8, 12, 15, 16, 25
19	192	4, 6, 8, 12, 15, 16
20	210	4, 6, 9, 12, 14, 15

Check your answers on p 147

SIMPLIFYING FRACTIONS I

To simplify (or 'cancel down') a fraction, divide the numerator *and* denominator by the *same* number. This number is called a *common factor*.

Notes:

* The *numerator* is the top number in a fraction.
* The *denominator* is the bottom number in a fraction.

Example A

Simplify $\dfrac{36}{48}$

$$\frac{36}{48} = \frac{3}{4} \quad \left[\begin{array}{l}\text{after dividing numerator and} \\ \text{denominator by 12}\end{array}\right]$$

Or this may be done in two or more steps:

$$\frac{36}{48} = \frac{18}{24} \quad \left[\begin{array}{l}\text{after dividing numerator and} \\ \text{denominator by 2}\end{array}\right]$$

$$= \frac{9}{12} \quad \left[\begin{array}{l}\text{after again dividing numerator and} \\ \text{denominator by 2}\end{array}\right]$$

$$= \frac{3}{4} \quad \left[\begin{array}{l}\text{after dividing numerator and} \\ \text{denominator by 3}\end{array}\right]$$

Note: $2 \times 2 \times 3 = 12$

Example B

Simplify $\dfrac{125}{225}$

$$\frac{125}{225} = \frac{25}{45} \quad \left[\begin{array}{l}\text{after dividing numerator and} \\ \text{denominator by 5}\end{array}\right]$$

$$= \frac{5}{9} \quad \left[\begin{array}{l}\text{after again dividing numerator and} \\ \text{denominator by 5}\end{array}\right]$$

Review exercise 1G *Simplify ('cancel down')*

Part i   *Simplify*

1	$\dfrac{8}{12}$	6	$\dfrac{15}{21}$	11	$\dfrac{28}{32}$	16	$\dfrac{14}{42}$	21	$\dfrac{36}{56}$
2	$\dfrac{10}{14}$	7	$\dfrac{20}{24}$	12	$\dfrac{22}{33}$	17	$\dfrac{30}{45}$	22	$\dfrac{48}{60}$
3	$\dfrac{6}{16}$	8	$\dfrac{20}{25}$	13	$\dfrac{15}{35}$	18	$\dfrac{42}{48}$	23	$\dfrac{52}{64}$
4	$\dfrac{9}{18}$	9	$\dfrac{12}{28}$	14	$\dfrac{32}{36}$	19	$\dfrac{36}{50}$	24	$\dfrac{21}{70}$
5	$\dfrac{15}{20}$	10	$\dfrac{9}{30}$	15	$\dfrac{16}{40}$	20	$\dfrac{25}{55}$	25	$\dfrac{32}{72}$

Part ii   *Simplify*

1	$\dfrac{75}{150}$	5	$\dfrac{125}{250}$	9	$\dfrac{30}{225}$	13	$\dfrac{125}{200}$	17	$\dfrac{175}{225}$
2	$\dfrac{75}{200}$	6	$\dfrac{125}{300}$	10	$\dfrac{40}{175}$	14	$\dfrac{375}{500}$	18	$\dfrac{225}{300}$
3	$\dfrac{75}{250}$	7	$\dfrac{125}{400}$	11	$\dfrac{45}{150}$	15	$\dfrac{275}{400}$	19	$\dfrac{425}{600}$
4	$\dfrac{75}{300}$	8	$\dfrac{125}{500}$	12	$\dfrac{60}{375}$	16	$\dfrac{100}{225}$	20	$\dfrac{325}{750}$

Check your answers on p 147

SIMPLIFYING FRACTIONS II

Example A

Simplify $\dfrac{900}{1500}$

$$\dfrac{900}{1500} = \dfrac{9}{15} \quad \left[\begin{array}{l}\text{after dividing numerator and} \\ \text{denominator by 100}\end{array}\right]$$

$$= \dfrac{3}{5} \quad \left[\begin{array}{l}\text{after dividing numerator and} \\ \text{denominator by 3}\end{array}\right]$$

Example B

Simplify $\dfrac{1400}{4000}$

$$\dfrac{1400}{4000} = \dfrac{14}{40} \quad \left[\begin{array}{l}\text{after dividing numerator and} \\ \text{denominator by 100}\end{array}\right]$$

$$= \dfrac{7}{20} \quad \left[\begin{array}{l}\text{after dividing numerator and} \\ \text{denominator by 2}\end{array}\right]$$

Review exercise 1H *Simplify ('cancel down')*

*Divide numerator **and** denominator by 10 or 100 or 1000 (whichever is appropriate). Then simplify further if possible.*

1	$\dfrac{30}{50}$	10	$\dfrac{120}{160}$	19	$\dfrac{400}{600}$	28	$\dfrac{1400}{2500}$
2	$\dfrac{40}{60}$	11	$\dfrac{100}{160}$	20	$\dfrac{450}{600}$	29	$\dfrac{2000}{2500}$
3	$\dfrac{60}{80}$	12	$\dfrac{60}{160}$	21	$\dfrac{540}{600}$	30	$\dfrac{1750}{2500}$
4	$\dfrac{50}{120}$	13	$\dfrac{200}{300}$	22	$\dfrac{600}{800}$	31	$\dfrac{2500}{3000}$
5	$\dfrac{80}{120}$	14	$\dfrac{120}{300}$	23	$\dfrac{750}{800}$	32	$\dfrac{500}{3000}$
6	$\dfrac{100}{120}$	15	$\dfrac{270}{300}$	24	$\dfrac{320}{800}$	33	$\dfrac{450}{3000}$
7	$\dfrac{130}{150}$	16	$\dfrac{300}{500}$	25	$\dfrac{1000}{1500}$	34	$\dfrac{1500}{4000}$
8	$\dfrac{100}{150}$	17	$\dfrac{450}{500}$	26	$\dfrac{800}{1500}$	35	$\dfrac{1200}{4000}$
9	$\dfrac{60}{150}$	18	$\dfrac{120}{500}$	27	$\dfrac{1250}{1500}$	36	$\dfrac{2750}{4000}$

Check your answers on p 148

SIMPLIFYING FRACTIONS III

Leave answers as *improper fractions*.

Example A

Simplify $\dfrac{175}{50}$

$$\dfrac{175}{50} = \dfrac{35}{10} \quad \left[\begin{array}{l}\text{after dividing numerator and}\\\text{denominator by 5}\end{array}\right]$$

$$= \dfrac{7}{2} \quad \left[\begin{array}{l}\text{after again dividing numerator and}\\\text{denominator by 5}\end{array}\right]$$

Example B

Simplify $\dfrac{400}{120}$

$$\dfrac{400}{120} = \dfrac{40}{12} \quad \left[\begin{array}{l}\text{after dividing numerator and}\\\text{denominator by 10}\end{array}\right]$$

$$= \dfrac{10}{3} \quad \left[\begin{array}{l}\text{after dividing numerator and}\\\text{denominator by 4}\end{array}\right]$$

A Review of Relevant Calculations

Review exercise 1I *Simplify ('cancel down')*

Leave answers as improper fractions

1 a $\dfrac{30}{20}$ b $\dfrac{50}{20}$ c $\dfrac{75}{20}$ d $\dfrac{85}{20}$

2 a $\dfrac{100}{8}$ b $\dfrac{150}{8}$ c $\dfrac{300}{8}$ d $\dfrac{750}{8}$

3 a $\dfrac{150}{12}$ b $\dfrac{350}{12}$ c $\dfrac{500}{12}$ d $\dfrac{1000}{12}$

4 a $\dfrac{100}{40}$ b $\dfrac{300}{40}$ c $\dfrac{380}{40}$ d $\dfrac{550}{40}$

5 a $\dfrac{70}{50}$ b $\dfrac{75}{50}$ c $\dfrac{120}{50}$ d $\dfrac{125}{50}$

6 a $\dfrac{80}{60}$ b $\dfrac{150}{60}$ c $\dfrac{750}{60}$ d $\dfrac{1000}{60}$

7 a $\dfrac{100}{80}$ b $\dfrac{200}{80}$ c $\dfrac{550}{80}$ d $\dfrac{1000}{80}$

8 a $\dfrac{180}{120}$ b $\dfrac{200}{120}$ c $\dfrac{300}{120}$ d $\dfrac{450}{120}$

9 a $\dfrac{200}{125}$ b $\dfrac{300}{125}$ c $\dfrac{800}{125}$ d $\dfrac{900}{125}$

10 a $\dfrac{150}{125}$ b $\dfrac{350}{125}$ c $\dfrac{550}{125}$ d $\dfrac{950}{125}$

11 a $\dfrac{180}{150}$ b $\dfrac{225}{150}$ c $\dfrac{400}{150}$ d $\dfrac{950}{150}$

12 a $\dfrac{800}{250}$ b $\dfrac{900}{250}$ c $\dfrac{1200}{250}$ d $\dfrac{1800}{250}$

Check your answers on p 149

SIMPLIFYING FRACTIONS IV

To simplify a fraction involving decimals, multiply the fraction by $\frac{10}{10}$ or $\frac{100}{100}$, depending on whether the *higher* (or *equal*) number of decimal places is 1 d.p. (then multiply by $\frac{10}{10}$) or 2 d.p. (then multiply by $\frac{100}{100}$).

Note: d.p. stands for decimal place(s).

Example A

Simplify $\dfrac{0.4}{0.6}$

$0.4 \leftarrow 1$ d.p. $\quad\begin{bmatrix}\text{both numerator and} \\ \text{denominator have 1 d.p.}\end{bmatrix}$
$0.6 \leftarrow 1$ d.p.

$$\frac{0.4}{0.6} \times \frac{10}{10} = \frac{4}{6} = \frac{2}{3}$$

Example B

Simplify $\dfrac{0.35}{0.4}$

$0.35 \leftarrow 2$ d.p. $\quad\begin{bmatrix}\text{numerator has 2 d.p.;} \\ \text{denominator has 1 d.p.}\end{bmatrix}$
$0.4 \;\leftarrow 1$ d.p.

$$\frac{0.35}{0.4} \times \frac{100}{100} = \frac{35}{40} = \frac{7}{8}$$

Example C

Simplify $\dfrac{100}{2.5}$

$100 \leftarrow 0$ d.p. $\quad\begin{bmatrix}\text{numerator has 0 d.p.;} \\ \text{denominator has 1 d.p.}\end{bmatrix}$
$2.5 \leftarrow 1$ d.p.

$$\frac{100}{2.5} \times \frac{10}{10} = \frac{1000}{25} = \frac{200}{5} = \frac{40}{1} = 40$$

Example D

Simplify $\dfrac{0.07}{0.02}$

$0.07 \leftarrow 2$ d.p. $\quad\begin{bmatrix}\text{both numerator and} \\ \text{denominator have 2 d.p.}\end{bmatrix}$
$0.02 \leftarrow 2$ d.p.

$$\frac{0.07}{0.02} \times \frac{100}{100} = \frac{7}{2} \quad\begin{bmatrix}\text{leave answer as} \\ \text{an improper fraction}\end{bmatrix}$$

A Review of Relevant Calculations

Review exercise 1J *Simplify. Answers may be left as improper fractions, where these occur. However, $\frac{5}{1}$ (for example) should be written as just 5.*

1	$\dfrac{0.4}{0.5}$	9	$\dfrac{0.75}{0.3}$	17	$\dfrac{0.05}{0.04}$	25	$\dfrac{0.3}{0.6}$
2	$\dfrac{0.6}{0.8}$	10	$\dfrac{0.95}{0.4}$	18	$\dfrac{0.04}{0.06}$	26	$\dfrac{0.06}{0.08}$
3	$\dfrac{0.9}{0.6}$	11	$\dfrac{200}{2.5}$	19	$\dfrac{0.07}{0.01}$	27	$\dfrac{0.9}{0.1}$
4	$\dfrac{0.3}{0.7}$	12	$\dfrac{100}{1.5}$	20	$\dfrac{0.04}{0.08}$	28	$\dfrac{300}{2.5}$
5	$\dfrac{0.8}{0.4}$	13	$\dfrac{300}{1.5}$	21	$\dfrac{0.6}{0.4}$	29	$\dfrac{0.25}{0.4}$
6	$\dfrac{0.35}{0.5}$	14	$\dfrac{100}{4.5}$	22	$\dfrac{0.03}{0.09}$	30	$\dfrac{0.05}{0.02}$
7	$\dfrac{0.45}{0.2}$	15	$\dfrac{500}{5.5}$	23	$\dfrac{0.15}{0.2}$	31	$\dfrac{0.75}{0.5}$
8	$\dfrac{0.55}{0.1}$	16	$\dfrac{0.09}{0.02}$	24	$\dfrac{200}{1.5}$	32	$\dfrac{100}{3.5}$

Check your answers on p 150

ROUNDING OFF DECIMAL NUMBERS

ROUNDING OFF TO *ONE* DECIMAL PLACE

Method If the *second* decimal place is *5 or more*, then *add 1* to the first decimal place. If the second decimal place is *less than 5*, then *leave* the first decimal place as it is.

Example A

Write correct to one decimal place

a	0.62	b	1.75	c	3.49
a	*0.6 ② ≈ 0.6*	b	*1.7 ⑤ ≈ 1.8*	c	*3.4 ⑨ ≈ 3.5*

Note: The symbol ≈ stands for *is approximately equal to*.

ROUNDING OFF TO *TWO* DECIMAL PLACES

Method If the *third* decimal place is *5 or more*, then *add 1* to the second decimal place. If the third decimal place is *less than 5*, then *leave* the second decimal place as it is.

Example B

Write correct to two decimal places

a	0.827	b	0.694	c	2.145
a	*0.82 ⑦ ≈ 0.83*	b	*0.69 ④ ≈ 0.69*	c	*2.14 ⑤ ≈ 2.15*

Review exercise 1K *Rounding off*

Part i *Write each number correct to **one** decimal place.*

1	0.93	5	0.58	9	2.37	13	1.06
2	0.47	6	0.96	10	1.09	14	2.98
3	0.85	7	1.57	11	0.16	15	1.02
4	0.69	8	1.22	12	2.65	16	0.75

Part ii *Write each number correct to **two** decimal places.*

1	0.333	5	0.142	9	2.714	13	0.625
2	1.667	6	0.125	10	1.285	14	0.777
3	0.875	7	0.916	11	0.636	15	2.428
4	0.833	8	1.571	12	0.222	16	1.857

Check your answers on p 150

Nursing Calculations

FRACTION TO A DECIMAL I

Some fractions have *exact* decimal equivalents; for example $\frac{1}{2}$ is exactly equal to 0.5. Other fractions have only *approximate* decimal equivalents; for example $\frac{2}{3}$ is approximately equal to 0.67. The fractions in this review exercise have *exact* decimal equivalents.

Method   Divide the numerator by the denominator.

Example A

Change $\dfrac{2}{5}$ to a decimal.

$5\overline{)2.0}$ ← Write as many zeros
$\underline{0.4}$ as you need

$\therefore \dfrac{2}{5} = 0.4$

Example B

Change $\dfrac{3}{8}$ to a decimal.

$8\overline{)3.0^6 0^4 0}$ ← Write as many zeros
$\underline{0.3\ 7\ 5}$ as you need

$\therefore \dfrac{3}{8} = 0.375$

Example C

Change $\dfrac{3}{20}$ to a decimal.

$10\overline{)3}$ 　⎡divided by 10
$2\overline{)0.3^1 0}$ 　and then 2
$\underline{0.1\ 5}$ 　since $10 \times 2 = 20$⎦

or $\dfrac{3}{20} = \dfrac{15}{100}$
　　　　$= 0.15$

Example D

Change $\dfrac{14}{25}$ to a decimal.

$5\overline{)14.^4 0}$ 　⎡divided by 5
$5\overline{)2.8^3 0}$ 　and then 5 again
$\underline{0.5\ 6}$ 　since $5 \times 5 = 25$⎦

or $\dfrac{14}{25} = \dfrac{56}{100}$
　　　　$= 0.56$

Review exercise 1L *Fraction to a decimal I*

Change each fraction to a decimal. All of these fractions have exact decimal equivalents. Refer to Examples A and B.

1 $\dfrac{1}{2}$ 3 $\dfrac{3}{4}$ 5 $\dfrac{3}{5}$ 7 $\dfrac{1}{8}$

2 $\dfrac{1}{4}$ 4 $\dfrac{1}{5}$ 6 $\dfrac{4}{5}$ 8 $\dfrac{7}{8}$

All of these fractions have exact decimal equivalents. Refer to Examples C and D.

9 $\dfrac{1}{20}$ 13 $\dfrac{1}{25}$ 17 $\dfrac{1}{40}$ 21 $\dfrac{1}{50}$

10 $\dfrac{7}{20}$ 14 $\dfrac{8}{25}$ 18 $\dfrac{9}{40}$ 22 $\dfrac{7}{50}$

11 $\dfrac{13}{20}$ 15 $\dfrac{17}{25}$ 19 $\dfrac{11}{40}$ 23 $\dfrac{21}{50}$

12 $\dfrac{19}{20}$ 16 $\dfrac{22}{25}$ 20 $\dfrac{27}{40}$ 24 $\dfrac{43}{50}$

Check your answers on p 151

FRACTION TO A DECIMAL II

The fractions in this review exercise have only approximate decimal equivalents.

Note: d.p. stands for decimal place(s).

Example A

Change $\dfrac{4}{7}$ to a decimal correct to 1 d.p.

$$7\overline{)4.0^50} \quad \leftarrow \text{Use 2 zeros}$$

0.5⑦ The second d.p. is 5 or more, therefore add 1 to the first d.p.

$\therefore \dfrac{4}{7} \approx 0.6$

Note: The symbol $\approx$ stands for is approximately equal to.

Example B

Change $\dfrac{5}{6}$ to a decimal correct to 2 d.p.

$$6\overline{)5.0^20^20} \quad \leftarrow \text{Use 3 zeros}$$

$0.8\,3\text{③}$ The third d.p. is less than 5, therefore leave second d.p. unchanged.

$\therefore \dfrac{5}{6} \approx 0.83$

Example C

Change $\dfrac{13}{60}$ to a decimal correct to 2 d.p.

$$10\overline{)13.0}$$
$$6\overline{)1.3^10^40}$$
$$\overline{\quad 0.2\,1\text{⑥}\quad}$$

$\begin{bmatrix} \text{divided by 10} \\ \text{and then 6} \\ \text{since } 10 \times 6 = 60 \end{bmatrix}$

$\therefore \dfrac{13}{60} \approx 0.22$

Review exercise 1M *Fraction to a decimal II*

Part i *Change each fraction to a decimal correct to **one** decimal place.*

1   $\dfrac{1}{3}$ 3 $\dfrac{2}{7}$ 5 $\dfrac{2}{9}$ 7 $\dfrac{6}{11}$

2   $\dfrac{5}{6}$ 4 $\dfrac{5}{7}$ 6 $\dfrac{3}{11}$ 8 $\dfrac{11}{12}$

Part ii *Change each fraction to a decimal correct to **two** decimal places.*

1   $\dfrac{2}{3}$ 3 $\dfrac{6}{7}$ 5 $\dfrac{8}{9}$ 7 $\dfrac{10}{11}$

2   $\dfrac{1}{6}$ 4 $\dfrac{4}{9}$ 6 $\dfrac{4}{11}$ 8 $\dfrac{5}{12}$

Check your answers on p 151

FRACTION TO A DECIMAL III

Note: d.p. stands for decimal place(s).

Example A

Calculate the value of $\dfrac{175}{6}$ to the nearest whole number.

$$\frac{175}{6} = 175 \div 6$$

$$\therefore \frac{175}{6} \approx 29.1 \Rightarrow 29$$

$$6{\overline{)}} \, 17^{5}5.^{1}0$$
$$ \; 2\,9.①$$

If the first d.p. is *5 or more*, then *add 1* to the whole number.

If the first d.p. is *less than 5*, then *leave* the whole number unchanged.

Example B

Calculate the value of $\dfrac{7}{6}$ correct to one decimal place.

$$\frac{7}{6} = 7 \div 6$$

$$\therefore \frac{7}{6} \approx 1.16 \Rightarrow 1.2$$

$$6{\overline{)}} \, 7.^{1}0^{4}0$$
$$ \; 1.1⑥$$

If the second d.p. is *5 or more*, then *add 1* to the first d.p.

If the second d.p. is *less than 5*, then *leave* the first d.p. unchanged.

Review exercise 1N *Fraction to a decimal III*

Part i *Calculate the value of each fraction to the nearest whole number.*
Refer to Example A.

1	$\dfrac{100}{3}$	5	$\dfrac{75}{4}$	9	$\dfrac{125}{6}$	13	$\dfrac{375}{8}$
2	$\dfrac{250}{3}$	6	$\dfrac{125}{4}$	10	$\dfrac{275}{6}$	14	$\dfrac{425}{8}$
3	$\dfrac{500}{3}$	7	$\dfrac{72}{5}$	11	$\dfrac{240}{7}$	15	$\dfrac{250}{9}$
4	$\dfrac{550}{3}$	8	$\dfrac{144}{5}$	12	$\dfrac{300}{7}$	16	$\dfrac{550}{9}$

Part ii *Calculate the value of each fraction correct to* **one** *decimal place.*
Refer to Example B.

1	$\dfrac{5}{3}$	5	$\dfrac{20}{7}$	9	$\dfrac{25}{8}$	13	$\dfrac{20}{9}$
2	$\dfrac{10}{3}$	6	$\dfrac{25}{7}$	10	$\dfrac{35}{8}$	14	$\dfrac{50}{9}$
3	$\dfrac{35}{6}$	7	$\dfrac{50}{7}$	11	$\dfrac{55}{8}$	15	$\dfrac{70}{9}$
4	$\dfrac{25}{6}$	8	$\dfrac{65}{7}$	12	$\dfrac{45}{8}$	16	$\dfrac{85}{9}$

Check your answers on p 151

MIXED NUMBERS AND IMPROPER FRACTIONS

A *mixed number* is partly a whole number and partly a fraction: e.g.
$3\frac{1}{2}$. In an *improper fraction*, the numerator is larger than the
denominator: e.g. $\dfrac{10}{7}$.

Example A

a **Change $\dfrac{17}{5}$ to a mixed number.**

$$\frac{17}{5} = 17 \div 5$$

$$= 3\tfrac{2}{5} \quad \leftarrow \text{remainder}$$
$\leftarrow$ same denominator as improper fraction

$$5)\underline{17}$$
$$3 + 2 \text{ remainder}$$

b **Change $\dfrac{115}{4}$ to a mixed number.**

$$\frac{115}{4} = 115 \div 4$$

$$= 28\tfrac{3}{4} \quad \leftarrow \text{remainder}$$
$\leftarrow$ same denominator as improper fraction

$$4)\underline{115}$$
$$28 + 3 \text{ remainder}$$

Example B

a **Change $8\frac{1}{4}$ to an improper fraction.**

$$8\frac{1}{4} = \frac{33}{4} \quad \leftarrow 8 \times 4 + 1 = 33$$
$\leftarrow$ same denominator as fraction in mixed number.

b **Change $20\frac{4}{5}$ to an improper fraction.**

$$20\frac{4}{5} = \frac{104}{5} \quad \leftarrow 20 \times 5 + 4 = 104$$
$\leftarrow$ same denominator as fraction in mixed number.

Review exercise 10 *Mixed numbers and improper fractions*

Part i *Change these improper fractions to mixed numbers.*

1	$\dfrac{5}{2}$	5	$\dfrac{29}{6}$	9	$\dfrac{51}{2}$	13	$\dfrac{95}{6}$	17	$\dfrac{133}{5}$
2	$\dfrac{11}{3}$	6	$\dfrac{36}{7}$	10	$\dfrac{65}{3}$	14	$\dfrac{101}{7}$	18	$\dfrac{143}{6}$
3	$\dfrac{17}{4}$	7	$\dfrac{37}{8}$	11	$\dfrac{71}{4}$	15	$\dfrac{113}{8}$	19	$\dfrac{157}{7}$
4	$\dfrac{22}{5}$	8	$\dfrac{49}{9}$	12	$\dfrac{86}{5}$	16	$\dfrac{125}{9}$	20	$\dfrac{166}{9}$

Part ii *Rewrite these mixed numbers as improper fractions.*

1	$1\frac{1}{2}$	5	$3\frac{1}{2}$	9	$11\frac{1}{6}$	13	$22\frac{1}{2}$	17	$30\frac{5}{6}$
2	$1\frac{1}{3}$	6	$4\frac{2}{3}$	10	$13\frac{2}{7}$	14	$24\frac{2}{3}$	18	$32\frac{4}{7}$
3	$1\frac{3}{4}$	7	$6\frac{1}{4}$	11	$16\frac{5}{8}$	15	$27\frac{3}{4}$	19	$35\frac{3}{8}$
4	$2\frac{3}{5}$	8	$9\frac{4}{5}$	12	$17\frac{2}{9}$	16	$29\frac{1}{5}$	20	$38\frac{5}{9}$

Check your answers on p 152

MULTIPLICATION OF FRACTIONS

There are two main methods of multiplying fractions. One method uses *cancelling before* multiplying the numerators and denominators; the other method uses *cancelling after* multiplying the numerators and denominators. We recommend the first method as this keeps the numbers smaller in the working out. Both methods are shown in Example B.

Example A

Multiply $\frac{2}{5} \times \frac{4}{7}$

Note: These fractions cannot be cancelled before multiplying.

$$\frac{2}{5} \times \frac{4}{7} = \frac{2 \times 4}{5 \times 7}$$

$$= \frac{8}{35} \quad \begin{bmatrix} \text{this fraction cannot} \\ \text{be simplified} \end{bmatrix}$$

Example B

Simplify $\frac{4}{9} \times \frac{21}{5}$

$$\frac{4}{\underset{3}{\cancel{9}}} \times \frac{\overset{7}{\cancel{21}}}{5} = \frac{4 \times 7}{3 \times 5}$$

note cancelling across by 3

$$= \frac{28}{15}$$

change to a mixed number

$$= 1\frac{13}{15}$$

answer may be greater than 1

$$\frac{4}{9} \times \frac{21}{5} = \frac{4 \times 21}{9 \times 5} = \frac{84}{45}$$

divide numerator and denominator by 3

$$= \frac{28}{15}$$

change to a mixed number

$$= 1\frac{13}{15}$$

answer may be greater than 1

Example C

Simplify $\frac{9}{10} \times \frac{8}{15}$

$$\frac{\overset{3}{\cancel{9}}}{\underset{5}{\cancel{10}}} \times \frac{\overset{4}{\cancel{8}}}{\underset{5}{\cancel{15}}} = \frac{3 \times 4}{5 \times 5} \quad \begin{bmatrix} \text{note cancelling across} \\ \text{by 3 and by 2} \end{bmatrix}$$

$$= \frac{12}{25}$$

Review exercise 1P *Multiplication of fractions*

Multiply these fractions. Simplify your answer where possible.

1 $\dfrac{1}{2} \times \dfrac{2}{5}$

2 $\dfrac{1}{3} \times \dfrac{5}{8}$

3 $\dfrac{2}{3} \times \dfrac{5}{6}$

4 $\dfrac{1}{4} \times \dfrac{2}{3}$

5 $\dfrac{3}{4} \times \dfrac{20}{9}$

6 $\dfrac{1}{5} \times \dfrac{3}{10}$

7 $\dfrac{2}{5} \times \dfrac{3}{2}$

8 $\dfrac{3}{5} \times \dfrac{3}{4}$

9 $\dfrac{4}{5} \times \dfrac{25}{24}$

10 $\dfrac{1}{6} \times \dfrac{9}{10}$

11 $\dfrac{5}{6} \times \dfrac{8}{15}$

12 $\dfrac{1}{7} \times \dfrac{7}{18}$

13 $\dfrac{2}{7} \times \dfrac{11}{12}$

14 $\dfrac{3}{7} \times \dfrac{1}{20}$

15 $\dfrac{4}{7} \times \dfrac{5}{3}$

16 $\dfrac{5}{7} \times \dfrac{12}{25}$

17 $\dfrac{6}{7} \times \dfrac{5}{24}$

18 $\dfrac{1}{8} \times \dfrac{1}{2}$

19 $\dfrac{3}{8} \times \dfrac{12}{5}$

20 $\dfrac{5}{8} \times \dfrac{9}{20}$

21 $\dfrac{7}{8} \times \dfrac{8}{7}$

22 $\dfrac{1}{9} \times \dfrac{1}{15}$

23 $\dfrac{2}{9} \times \dfrac{7}{4}$

24 $\dfrac{4}{9} \times \dfrac{5}{12}$

25 $\dfrac{5}{9} \times \dfrac{21}{25}$

26 $\dfrac{7}{9} \times \dfrac{9}{16}$

27 $\dfrac{8}{9} \times \dfrac{1}{6}$

28 $\dfrac{1}{10} \times \dfrac{15}{8}$

29 $\dfrac{3}{10} \times \dfrac{4}{9}$

30 $\dfrac{7}{10} \times \dfrac{2}{7}$

Check your answers on p 153

MULTIPLICATION OF A FRACTION BY A WHOLE NUMBER

Example A

Multiply $\dfrac{5}{4} \times 6$. Simplify if possible. Write your answer as a fraction, a mixed number, or a whole number.

$$Simplify\ \frac{5}{4} \times 6 = \frac{5}{4} \times \frac{6}{1}$$

$$= \frac{30}{4} \quad \begin{bmatrix} \text{Divide numerator and} \\ \text{denominator by 2} \end{bmatrix}$$

$$= \frac{15}{2} \quad \begin{bmatrix} \text{Change to a} \\ \text{mixed number} \end{bmatrix}$$

$$= 7\frac{1}{2}$$

Example B

Multiply $\dfrac{150}{125} \times 2$. Write your answer as a decimal number.

$$\frac{150}{125} \times 2 = \frac{150}{125} \times \frac{2}{1}$$

$$= \frac{300}{125} \quad \begin{bmatrix} \text{Divide numerator and} \\ \text{denominator by 5} \end{bmatrix}$$

$$= \frac{60}{25} \quad \begin{bmatrix} \text{Again divide numerator and} \\ \text{denominator by 5} \end{bmatrix}$$

$$= \frac{12}{5} \quad [\text{Divide 12 by 5}]$$

$$= 2.4$$

Review exercise 1Q *Multiply these fractions and whole numbers*

Part i *Multiply. Simplify where possible. Write each answer as a fraction, a mixed number, or a whole number.*

1 $\frac{3}{4} \times 5$

2 $\frac{2}{5} \times 3$

3 $\frac{2}{3} \times 6$

4 $\frac{5}{3} \times 4$

5 $\frac{3}{5} \times 10$

6 $\frac{2}{7} \times 3$

7 $\frac{3}{4} \times 6$

8 $\frac{5}{8} \times 3$

9 $\frac{4}{5} \times 5$

10 $\frac{5}{6} \times 4$

11 $\frac{2}{3} \times 5$

12 $\frac{3}{10} \times 2$

Part ii *Multiply. Write each answer as a decimal number, or as a whole number, where this occurs.*

1 $\frac{7}{4} \times 2$

2 $\frac{6}{10} \times 2$

3 $\frac{3}{10} \times 2$

4 $\frac{7}{20} \times 2$

5 $\frac{25}{20} \times 2$

6 $\frac{18}{50} \times 5$

7 $\frac{90}{50} \times 2$

8 $\frac{60}{80} \times 5$

9 $\frac{32}{40} \times 2$

10 $\frac{35}{50} \times 4$

11 $\frac{45}{25} \times 5$

12 $\frac{55}{50} \times 4$

24-HOUR TIME

Example A *Convert to 24-hour time*

a **8:45 am**
b **4:20 pm**
a 8:45 am = 08:45 hours
b 4:20 pm = 4:20 + 12:00 = 16:20 hours

Note: In practice, the colons [:] are usually omitted. So 08:45 hours would simply be written as 0845 hours and 16:20 hours would be written as 1620 hours.

Example B *Convert to am/pm time*

a **1150 hours**
b **2015 hours**
a 1150 hours = 11:50 am
b 2015 hours = 2015 − 1200 = 8:15 pm

Example C

What is the time 6 hours after 1915 hours on a Thursday? Give time and day.

1915 hours + 6 hr 00 mins = 2515 hours

But there are only 24 hours in a day

2515 hours − 2400 = 0115 hours Friday

Note: noon = 1200 hours; midnight = 2400 hours.

Review exercise 1R *24-hour time*

Part i *Convert to 24-hour time.*

1	9:10 am	5	4:00 am	9	6:20 am
2	8:40 pm	6	3:25 pm	10	5:35 pm
3	2:30 am	7	12:55 pm	11	7:45 am
4	11:05 am	8	1:15 pm	12	10:50 pm

Part ii *Convert to am/pm time.*

1	1935 hours	5	1305 hours	9	2315 hours
2	2230 hours	6	1745 hours	10	0510 hours
3	0105 hours	7	2125 hours	11	1220 hours
4	0200 hours	8	0640 hours	12	1450 hours

Part iii *Calculate the finishing times. Give answers in 24-hour time and also give the day.*

1 8 hours after 0945 hours Monday

2 7 hours after 2230 hours Thursday

3 10 hours after 1015 hours Saturday

4 11 hours after 1700 hours Tuesday

5 9 hours after 2025 hours Sunday

6 12 hours after 0640 hours Wednesday

7 12 hours after 1220 hours Friday

8 14 hours after 0510 hours Thursday

Check your answers on p 154

24-HOUR TIME

am/pm time	24-hour time (hours)	am/pm time	24-hour time (hours)
1 am	0100	1 pm	1300
2 am	0200	2 pm	1400
3 am	0300	3 pm	1500
4 am	0400	4 pm	1600
5 am	0500	5 pm	1700
6 am	0600	6 pm	1800
7 am	0700	7 pm	1900
8 am	0800	8 pm	2000
9 am	0900	9 pm	2100
10 am	1000	10 pm	2200
11 am	1100	11 pm	2300
12 noon	1200	12 midnight	2400

Note: You may also see midnight written as 0000 hours. One minute past midnight is 0001.

Dosages of oral medications 2

Drugs may be administered via several routes, including by injection, by intravenous infusion, or orally. The first medications that a nursing student will administer to patients are usually oral medications.

Skills covered in this chapter include:

- calculating the actual dose required for an oral medication based on the prescription
- identifying the best combination of tablets required for specific prescriptions, so as few tablets as possible are used
- calculating the amount of liquid medication in a specific volume
- interpreting the information on a medication chart and medication labels to accurately calculate dosages.

WHAT YOU NEED TO KNOW

Oral dosages may be in the form of tablets or capsules or in liquid form.

A whole tablet is *always* preferable to a broken tablet because, unless a tablet is broken accurately, the dose will not be exact. If it is necessary to break a tablet or capsule, check the manufacturer's guidelines or check with the pharmacist to ensure it is acceptable to do so, as some should *never* be broken.

Many oral medications are available in liquid form. The liquid may be a syrup, an elixir, a solution or a suspension.

Important: Suspensions must be shaken thoroughly before measuring the required volume.

Check that stock strength and the strength required are given in the *same* unit in a particular calculation (i.e. *both* strengths in grams or milligrams or micrograms).

Important: If in **any** doubt about the answer to a calculation, then ask a supervisor to check your calculation.

Refer to prelim page ix for explanations of abbreviations.

CHAPTER CONTENTS

CALCULATING DOSAGES OF TABLETS AND CAPSULES

Example A *How many 50 mg tablets of atenolol should be given for a dose of atenolol 75 mg?*

$$\text{Volume required} = \frac{\text{Strength required}}{\text{Stock strength}} \times [\text{Volume of stock solution}]$$

The formula can be abbreviated to:

$$VR = \frac{SR}{SS} \times VS$$

$$= \frac{75 \text{ mg}}{50 \text{ mg}} \times 1 \text{ tablet}$$

$$= \frac{3}{2} \text{ tablets}$$

$$= 1\frac{1}{2} \text{ tablets}$$

Note: In the case of tablets, 'Volume required' refers to the number of tablets.

Nursing Calculations

Example B *A patient is prescribed 0.25 mg of digoxin, orally (PO) at 0800 hrs. The digoxin available is in tablets containing 125 micrograms. How many of these tablets should the patient receive?*

Note: First step– change both strengths to the same units.

$$0.25 \text{ mg} = 250 \text{ micrograms}$$

$$\text{Volume required} = \frac{\text{Strength required}}{\text{Stock strength}} \times [\text{Volume of stock solution}]$$

The formula can be abbreviated to:

$$VR = \frac{SR}{SS} \times VS$$

$$= \frac{250 \text{ micrograms}}{125 \text{ micrograms}} \times 1 \text{ tablet}$$

$$= \frac{2}{1} \text{ tablets}$$

$$= 2 \text{ tablets}$$

If you are having difficulty simplifying the fractions in these examples, then refer to Review exercises 1H and 1I in Chapter 1.

Dosages of Oral Medications

Exercise 2A

1 A patient is prescribed paracetamol 1 g, orally. The stock available is 500 mg capsules. Calculate the number of capsules required.

2 Prescribed: codeine 15 mg, PO, 1200 hrs. Stock on hand: codeine 30 mg tablets. How many tablets should be administered to the patient?

3 A patient is prescribed furosemide (frusemide) 60 mg, orally. In the ward are 40 mg tablets. How many tablets should be given?

4 How many 30 mg tablets of codeine are needed for a dose of 0.06 g?

5 750 mg of ciprofloxacin is required. The available tablets are of strength 500 mg. How many tablets should be given?

6 A patient is prescribed 150 mg of soluble aspirin at 1000 hrs. On hand are 300 mg tablets. What number should be given?

7 450 mg of soluble aspirin is prescribed. Stock available is 300 mg tablets. How many tablets should the patient receive?

8 25 mg captopril PO is prescribed. How many 50 mg tablets should be given?

9 The stock available in the unit is diazepam 5 mg tablets. How many tablets are to be administered if the prescription is diazepam 12.5 mg at 1400 hrs?

10 Digoxin 125 micrograms is prescribed at 0800 hrs. Tablets available are 0.25 mg. How many tablets should be given?

Check that you have used the **same unit of weight** through-out a calculation.
   Are **both** weights in grams (g)?
   or are **both** weights in milligrams (mg)?
   or are **both** weights in micrograms?

Check your answers on p 155

COMBINATIONS OF TABLETS

For some medications, tablets are available in different strengths. The tablets may be colour-coded to reduce the risk of error when dispensing.

Note: The *least* number of tablets is the best combination to be given to the patient.

Example *Choose the best combination of 1 mg, 2 mg, 5 mg or 10 mg tablets of warfarin for each dosage.*

The number of tablets should be as few as possible and only whole tablets may be used.

a **6 mg**   b **8 mg**   c **11 mg**   d **14 mg**

a 5 mg + 1 mg (2 tablets)
b 5 mg + 2 mg + 1 mg (3 tablets)
c 10 mg + 1 mg (2 tablets)
d 10 mg + 2 mg + 2 mg (3 tablets)

Exercise 2B *Choose the best combination of **whole** tablets for each prescription.*

The number of tablets should be as few as possible.

1   *Prescribed*: warfarin tablets
    Strengths available: 1 mg, 2 mg, 5 mg, 10 mg
    Dosages required: **a** 4 mg   **b** 9 mg   **c** 12 mg   **d** 15 mg

2   *Prescribed*: diazepam tablets
    Strengths available: 2 mg, 5 mg, 10 mg
    Dosages required: **a** 7 mg   **b** 9 mg   **c** 15 mg   **d** 20 mg

3   *Prescribed*: verapamil tablets
    Strengths available: 40 mg, 80 mg, 120 mg, 160 mg
    Dosages required: **a** 200 mg   **b** 240 mg   **c** 280 mg   **d** 320 mg

4   *Prescribed*: prazosin tablets
    Strengths available: 1 mg, 2 mg, 5 mg
    Dosages required: **a** 6 mg   **b** 8 mg   **c** 9 mg   **d** 11 mg

5   *Prescribed*: furosemide (frusemide) tablets
    Strengths available: 20 mg, 40 mg, 80 mg, 500 mg
    Dosages required: **a** 60 mg   **b** 100 mg   **c** 200 mg   **d** 560 mg

6   *Prescribed*: thioridazine tablets
    Strengths available: 10 mg, 25 mg, 50 mg, 100 mg
    Dosages required: **a** 35 mg   **b** 60 mg   **c** 75 mg   **d** 120 mg

---

Check your answers on p 155

STRENGTH OF SOLUTION ACCORDING TO VOLUME

Example *A syrup contains penicillin 125 mg/5 mL.* ★ *How many milligrams of penicillin are in the following volumes of the syrup?*

a	10 mL	b	15 mL	c	25 mL

a   Each 5 mL contains 125 mg penicillin

$$10\,mL \div 5\,mL = 2$$

$$2 \times 125\,mg = 250\,mg\ penicillin$$

b   Each 5 mL contains 125 mg penicillin

$$15\,mL \div 5\,mL = 3$$

$$3 \times 125\,mg = 375\,mg\ penicillin$$

c   Each 5 mL contains 125 mg penicillin

$$25\,mL \div 5\,mL = 5$$

$$5 \times 125\,mg = 625\,mg\ penicillin$$

★Note: 125 mg/5 mL means 125 mg *per* 5 mL.

Exercise 2C

1. A solution contains furosemide (frusemide) 10 mg per 1 mL. How many milligrams of frusemide are in
   a 2 mL   b 3 mL   c 5 mL of the solution?

2. A solution contains morphine hydrochloride 2 mg per mL. How many milligrams of morphine hydrochloride are in
   a 3 mL   b 5 mL   c 7 mL of the solution?

3. A solution contains morphine hydrochloride 40 mg/mL. How many milligrams of morphine hydrochloride are in
   a 2 mL   b 5 mL   c 10 mL of this solution?

4. A suspension contains phenytoin 125 mg per 5 mL. How many milligrams of phenytoin are in
   a 20 mL   b 30 mL   c 40 mL of the suspension?

5. A solution contains fluoxetine 20 mg/5 mL. How many milligrams of fluoxetine are in
   a 10 mL   b 25 mL   c 40 mL of the solution?

6. A suspension contains erythromycin 250 mg/5 mL. How many milligrams of erythromycin are in
   a 10 mL   b 20 mL   c 30 mL of the suspension?

7. A syrup contains chlorpromazine 25 mg per 5 mL. How many milligrams of chlorpromazine are in
   a 10 mL   b 30 mL   c 50 mL of the syrup?

8. A mixture contains penicillin 250 mg/5 mL. How many milligrams of penicillin are in
   a 15 mL   b 25 mL   c 35 mL of the mixture?

Check your answers on p 156

CALCULATING DOSAGES OF LIQUID MEDICATIONS

Example A *750 mg of erythromycin is to be given orally at 0700 hrs. Stock suspension contains 250 mg/5 mL. Calculate the volume to be given.*

$$\text{Volume required} = \frac{\text{Strength required}}{\text{Stock strength}} \times [\text{Volume of stock solution}]$$

$$= \frac{750 \text{ mg}}{250 \text{ mg}} \times 5 \text{ mL}$$

$$= \frac{750}{250} \times \frac{5}{1} \text{ mL}$$

$$= \frac{3}{1} \times \frac{5}{1} \text{ mL} \left[\text{after simplifying } \frac{750}{250} \right]$$

$$= 15 \text{ mL}$$

Example B *A patient is prescribed 800 mg of penicillin, PO. The stock available in the unit has a strength of 250 mg/5 mL. Calculate the volume required.*

The *volume required* formula can be abbreviated to:

$$\text{VR} = \frac{\text{SR}}{\text{SS}} \times \text{VS}$$

$$= \frac{800 \text{ mg}}{250 \text{ mg}} \times 5 \text{ mL}$$

$$= \frac{800}{250} \times \frac{5}{1} \text{ mL}$$

$$= \frac{16}{5} \times \frac{5}{1} \text{ mL} \left[\text{after simplifying } \frac{800}{250} \right]$$

$$= 16 \text{ mL}$$

If you are having difficulty simplifying the fractions in these examples, then refer to Review exercises 1H and 1I in Chapter 1.

Exercise 2D *You are given the prescribed dosage and the strength of stock available. Calculate the volume to be given.*

1   *Prescribed:* penicillin 500 mg
    Available: syrup 125 mg/5 mL

2   *Prescribed:* furosemide (frusemide) 40 mg
    Available: solution 10 mg/mL

3   *Prescribed:* morphine hydrochloride 100 mg
    Available: solution 40 mg/mL

4   *Prescribed:* paracetamol 180 mg
    Available: suspension 120 mg/5 mL

5   *Prescribed:* phenytoin 150 mg
    Available: suspension 125 mg/5 mL

6   *Prescribed:* erythromycin 1250 mg
    Available: suspension 250 mg/5 mL

7   *Prescribed:* fluoxetine 30 mg
    Available: solution 20 mg/5 mL

8   *Prescribed:* penicillin 1000 mg
    Available: mixture 250 mg/5 mL

9   *Prescribed:* chlorpromazine 35 mg
    Available: syrup 25 mg/5 mL

10 *Prescribed:* penicillin 1200 mg
    Available: mixture 250 mg/5 mL

11 *Prescribed:* erythromycin 800 mg
    Available: mixture 125 mg/5 mL

Check your answers on p 156

ORAL CALCULATIONS INVOLVING PRESCRIPTIONS AND MEDICATION LABELS

Exercise 2E *Read each prescription and medication label carefully.*

1   A patient is to be given their daily morning dose of oral ramipril. How many of these Tritace tablets should be given?

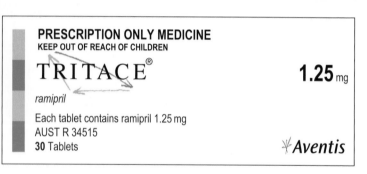

Regular medicines

Year 20 16		Date and month ⟶		2/3	3/3	4/3	5/3					
PRESCRIBER MUST ENTER administration times ◥												
Date 2/3	Medicine (print generic name) RAMIPRIL	Tick if slow release									Continue on discharge? Yes / No	
Route PO	Dose 2.5 mg MANE	Frequency and NOW enter times ⟶	0800	BG	KN	CM	BY				Dispense? Yes / No	Date:
Indication HYPERTENSION		Pharmacy									days Qty:	
Prescriber signature BCG	Print your name BLACK	Contact 46									Duration:	

PRESCRIPTION ONLY MEDICINE
KEEP OUT OF REACH OF CHILDREN

TRITACE®   **1.25** mg

ramipril

Each tablet contains ramipril 1.25 mg
AUST R 34515
30 Tablets   ⚘*Aventis*

2   How many Metronide tablets should be given for a dose in the
    following prescription of oral metronidazole?

Regular medicines

Date 20 16		Date and month →	10/1											
PRESCRIBER MUST ENTER administration times														
Date 20/1	Medicine (print generic name) METRONIDAZOLE	Tick if slow release	0800 PR											
Route PO	Dose 400 mg	Frequency and NOW enter times TDS →	1400 LL											
Indication INFECTION		Pharmacy	1400 LL											
Prescriber signature Singh	Print your name SINGH	Contact 762	2000											

Right column: Continue on discharge? Yes / No Dispense? Yes / No Duration: ___ days Qty: ___ Date: ___

PRESCRIPTION ONLY MEDICINE
KEEP OUT OF REACH OF CHILDREN

METRONIDE® 200

Metronidazole Tablets
21 TABLETS
Each tablet contains METRONIDAZOLE 200 mg
AUST R 65540

Check your answers on p 156

3 a How many mg of furosemide (frusemide) in

   i   1 mL

   ii 2 mL of Lasix oral solution?

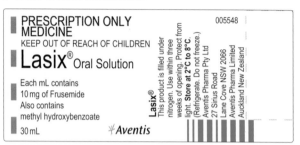

PRESCRIPTION ONLY MEDICINE

KEEP OUT OF REACH OF CHILDREN

Lasix® Oral Solution

Each mL contains
10 mg of Frusemide
Also contains
methyl hydroxybenzoate
30 mL

✳ *Aventis*

005548

Lasix®
This product is filled under nitrogen. Use within three weeks of opening. Protect from light. **Store at 2°C to 8°C.** (Refrigerate. Do not freeze.)
Aventis Pharma Pty Ltd
27 Sirius Road
Lane Cove NSW 2066
Aventis Pharma Limited
Auckland New Zealand

b Calculate the volume required for the dose in the prescription.

Regular medicines

Year 20 _16_ Date and month ⟶		4/2								Continue on discharge? Yes / No
PRESCRIBER MUST ENTER administration times ↘										Dispense? Yes / No
Date 4/2 Medicine (print generic name) FRUSEMIDE Tick if slow release	0800									Duration: ___ days Qty: ___
Route PO Dose 40 mg Frequency and NOW enter times ⟶ MANE										Date:
Indication HEART FAILURE Pharmacy LIQUID										
Prescriber signature NwG Print your name NwOJU Contact 961										

4 a How many mg of chlorpromazine in

   i   5 mL

   ii 10 mL of Largactil syrup?

PRESCRIPTION ONLY MEDICINE
KEEP OUT OF REACH OF CHILDREN

Largactil® Syrup

chlorpromazine hydrochloride

25 mg

Chlorpromazine oral solution
Each 5mL contains 25mg
chlorpromazine hydrochloride

100mL syrup   ✳ *Aventis*

Largactil® Syrup
Contact with the skin should be avoided by those
handling Largactil preparations to minimise the
risk of dermatitis.

This medicine may cause drowsiness and may
increase the effects of alcohol. If affected, do not
drive or operate machinery.

DOSAGE: As directed by physician.
Store below 25°C. Protect from light.

Aventis Pharma Pty Ltd
27 Sirius Road
Lane Cove NSW 2066
Australia

005905

---

b Calculate the volume required for a dose in the prescription.

Regular medicines

Year 20 16		Date and month ➝	15/1									
PRESCRIBER MUST ENTER administration times ➜												
Date 15/1	Medicine (print generic name) CHLORPROMAZINE	Tick if slow release										
		0800									Continue on discharge? Yes / No	
Route Po	Dose 40 mg Frequency and NOW enter times TDS	1400									Dispense? Yes / No	Date:
Indication AGITATION	Pharmacy LIQUID										days Qty:	
Prescriber signature TZowski	Print your name ZOWSKI	Contact 588	2000								Duration:	

CHAPTER 2 REVISION

1   A patient is prescribed penicillin 500 mg orally at 1700 hrs. In the ward are 250 mg capsules. What number should be given?

2   12.5 mg of captopril is prescribed for hypertension. On hand are tablets with a strength of 25 mg. How many tablets should be given?

3   How many 30 mg tablets of codeine should be given for a prescription of codeine 45 mg?

4   Choose the best combination of 1 mg, 2 mg, 5 mg and 10 mg tablets of warfarin for each of these dosages:
    a 3 mg   b 7 mg   c 13 mg   d 16 mg

5   Many oral medications in liquid form are suspensions. What must be done to those medications before measuring out the required volume?

6   A solution contains furosemide (frusemide) 10 mg/mL. How many milligrams of furosemide are in
    a 5 mL   b 10 mL   c 25 mL of the solution?

7   A suspension contains erythromycin 250 mg per 5 mL. How many milligrams of erythromycin are in
    a 15 mL   b 25 mL   c 35 mL of the suspension?

8   A patient is prescribed 750 mg of erythromycin, orally. Calculate the volume required if the suspension on hand has a strength of 250 mg/5 mL.

9   Paracetamol 750 mg is to be given at 1500 hrs as a syrup. The available stock contains 150 mg per 5 mL. Calculate the volume of syrup to be given.

10 A patient is prescribed penicillin 400 mg, orally, at 1600 hrs. Stock syrup has a strength of 125 mg/5 mL. What volume should be given?

11 Flucloxacillin 375 mg is prescribed. Stock syrup contains 125 mg per 5 mL. What volume of syrup should the patient be given?

12 Furosemide (frusemide) 125 mg at 0200 hrs is prescribed. Stock solution is 50 mg/mL. What volume of solution should be given?

Check your answers on p 157

Dosages of medications for injection

Correct measurement of dosages of medications for injection is essential. An overdose can be dangerous; too low a dose may result in a medication being ineffective.

In this chapter you will be shown how to calculate the volume of medication to be drawn up in a syringe, to be given by injection.

WHAT YOU NEED TO KNOW

The number of decimal places in each answer should relate to the graduations on the syringe being used. Syringes with a capacity of more than 1 mL are usually graduated in tenths or fifths of a millilitre: so for volumes *greater* than 1 mL calculate answers to *one* decimal place. Syringes with a capacity of 1 mL or less are often graduated in hundredths of a millilitre: so for volumes *less* than 1 mL calculate answers to *two* decimal places.

Remember:

- Give answers greater than 1 mL correct to one decimal place
- Give answers less than 1 mL correct to two decimal places
- If the next decimal place is 5 or more, add one to the previous digit
- Check that stock strength and the strength required are given in the *same* units in a particular calculation (i.e. *both* strengths in grams or milligrams or micrograms).

Important: If in **any** doubt about the answer to a calculation, then ask a supervisor to check your work.

Refer to prelim page ix for explanations of abbreviations.

CHAPTER CONTENTS

Dosages of Medications for Injection

ESTIMATING THE VOLUME FOR INJECTION

It is important to learn how to estimate an answer *before* beginning to work out the actual answer.

Example A *Pethidine 75 mg is to be given by IM injection. Stock ampoules of pethidine contain 100 mg in 2 mL. Is the volume to be drawn up for injection equal to 2 mL, less than 2 mL, or more than 2 mL?*

A stock ampoule contains 100 mg of pethidine.
Volume of ampoule = 2 mL
75 mg (prescribed) is *less than* 100 mg (ampoule).
Therefore, volume to be drawn up is *less than* 2 mL.

Example B *Vancomycin 1200 mg is prescribed at 2400 hrs. Stock vials contain vancomycin 1 g in 10 mL (once diluted). Is the volume of stock required for injection equal to 10 mL, less than 10 mL, or more than 10 mL?*

A stock vial contains 1 g of vancomycin.
1 g = 1 gram = 1000 mg
Volume of vial = 10 mL
1200 mg (prescribed) is *more than* 1000 mg (vial).
Therefore, volume required is *more than* 10 mL.

Example C *A patient is to be given 12 000 units of Calciparine at 0600 hrs. Available ampoules contain 25 000 units in 1 mL. Should the volume to be drawn up for injection be equal to 1 mL, less than 1 mL, or more than 1 mL?*

A stock ampoule contains 25 000 units.
Volume of ampoule = 1 mL
12 000 units (prescribed) is *less than* 25 000 units (ampoule).
Therefore, volume to be drawn up is *less than* 1 mL.

Exercise 3A *Choose the correct answer to each problem.*

The answer will be equal to, less than, or more than the volume of the stock ampoule or vial.

1   An injection of morphine 9 mg is prescribed. A stock ampoule contains morphine 15 mg in 1 mL. The volume to be drawn up for injection will be: equal to 1 mL/less than 1 mL/more than 1 mL.

2   A patient is to receive an injection of ondansetron 6 mg. Stock ampoules contain ondansetron 4 mg in 2 mL. The volume to be drawn up for injection is: equal to 2 mL/less than 2 mL/more than 2 mL.

3   Furosemide (frusemide) 80 mg is prescribed. Ampoules contain furosemide 250 mg/5 mL. The volume required for injection is: equal to 5 mL/less than 5 mL/more than 5 mL.

4   Benzylpenicillin 1.2 g is prescribed. Stock vials contain 600 mg in 2 mL, when diluted. The volume of stock required is: equal to 2 mL/less than 2 mL/more than 2 mL.

5   A patient is prescribed flucloxacillin 1000 mg, IV. If stock ampoules contain 1 g in 10 mL, once diluted, then the amount of stock solution to be drawn up will be: equal to 10 mL/less than 10 mL/more than 10 mL.

6   On hand are digoxin ampoules containing 500 micrograms in 2 mL. An injection of 225 micrograms is prescribed. The volume required is: equal to 2 mL/less than 2 mL/more than 2 mL.

7   Heparin is available at a strength of 1000 units per mL. The volume needed to give 1250 units is: equal to 1 mL/less than 1 mL/more than 1 mL.

8   Diazepam 15 mg is to be given by IV injection. Stock ampoules contain 10 mg in 2 mL. The volume to be drawn up is: equal to 2 mL/less than 2 mL/more than 2 mL.

Think carefully about each answer in the exercises that follow in this chapter. Should the volume to be drawn up for injection be equal to, less than, or more than the volume of the stock ampoule?

Check your answers on p 158

CALCULATING VOLUMES OF DOSAGES FOR INJECTION

Example A *A patient is prescribed furosemide (frusemide) 60 mg, IV. Ampoules contain furosemide 80 mg in 2 mL. Calculate the volume required for injection.*

$$\text{Volume required} = \frac{\text{Strength required}}{\text{Stock strength}} \times [\text{Volume of stock solution}]$$

$$= \frac{60\,\text{mg}}{80\,\text{mg}} \times 2\,\text{mL}$$

$$= \frac{60}{80} \times \frac{2}{1}\,\text{mL}$$

$$= \frac{3}{2}\,\text{mL}$$

$$= 1.5\,\text{mL}$$

Example B *An injection of digoxin 175 micrograms is prescribed. Stock on hand is digoxin 500 micrograms in 2 mL. What volume of stock solution should be given?*

The *volume required* formula can be abbreviated to:

$$VR = \frac{SR}{SS} \times VS$$

$$= \frac{175\,\text{micrograms}}{500\,\text{micrograms}} \times 2\,\text{mL}$$

$$= \frac{175}{500} \times \frac{2}{1}\,\text{mL}$$

$$= \frac{7}{10}\,\text{mL}$$

$$= 0.7\,\text{mL}$$

If you are having difficulty simplifying the fractions in these examples, then refer to Review exercises 1H and 1I in Chapter 1.

Nursing Calculations

Exercise 3B

1 An injection of morphine 8 mg is required. Ampoules on hand contain 10 mg in 1 mL. What volume should be drawn up for injection?

2 Digoxin ampoules on hand contain 500 micrograms in 2 mL. What volume is needed to administer 350 micrograms?

3 A child is prescribed 9 mg of gentamicin by IM injection at 0900 hrs. Stock ampoules contain 20 mg in 2 mL. What volume is needed for the injection?

4 A patient is to be given flucloxacillin 250 mg by injection. Stock vials contain 1 g in 10 mL, after dilution. Calculate the required volume.

5 Stock heparin has a strength of 5000 units per mL. What volume must be drawn up to give 6500 units subcut?

6 Pethidine 85 mg is to be given IM. Stock ampoules contain pethidine 100 mg in 2 mL. Calculate the volume of stock required.

7 A patient is to receive an injection of gentamicin 60 mg IM at 0200 hrs. Ampoules on hand contain 80 mg/2 mL. Calculate the volume required.

8 A patient is prescribed naloxone 0.6 mg IV stat. Stock ampoules contain 0.4 mg/2 mL. What volume should be drawn up for injection?

Think about each answer. Does it make sense? Is it ridiculously large?

Check your answers on p 158

Exercise 3C

1 Vancomycin 500 mg is prescribed at 2000 hrs. Stock on hand contains 1 g in 10 mL, once diluted. What volume is required?

2 A patient is to receive an IV dose of gentamicin 160 mg. Stock ampoules contain 100 mg in 2 mL. Calculate the volume to be drawn up for injection.

3 How much morphine solution must be withdrawn for a 7.5 mg dose if a stock ampoule contains 15 mg in 1 mL?

4 A patient is prescribed 200 mg of furosemide (frusemide) at 1000 hrs. Stock is 250 mg in 5 mL. Calculate the volume that is needed for injection.

5 Heparin is available at a strength of 5000 units/5 mL. What volume is needed to give 800 units?

6 Phenobarbitone 40 mg has been prescribed. Stock ampoules contain 200 mg/mL. What volume should be given?

7 A patient is prescribed pethidine 65 mg stat. Stock ampoules of pethidine contain 100 mg in 2 mL. Calculate the volume to be drawn up for injection.

8 A patient is to be given ranitidine 40 mg IV at 1230 hrs. Stock ampoules have a strength of 50 mg per 2 mL. What volume of stock should be injected?

9 Morphine 5.5 mg at 1600 hrs is prescribed. Stock ampoules contain 10 mg/mL. What volume should be drawn up for injection?

Check your answers on p 158

Exercise 3D *Calculate the volume of stock to be drawn up for injection.*

1   Pethidine 60 mg stat is prescribed. Stock ampoules contain 100 mg in 2 mL.

2   An adult is prescribed metoclopramide 15 mg, for nausea. On hand are ampoules containing 10 mg/mL.

3   A patient is prescribed erythromycin 250 mg IV at 1430 hrs. Stock on hand contains 1 g in 10 mL, once diluted.

4   Tramadol hydrochloride 80 mg is required. Available stock contains 100 mg in 2 mL.

5   A patient is prescribed benzylpenicillin 800 mg at 0830 hrs. On hand is benzylpenicillin 1.2 g in 6 mL.

6   An adult patient with tuberculosis is to be given 500 mg of capreomycin every second day by IM injection. Stock on hand contains 1 g in 3 mL.

7   Digoxin ampoules on hand contain 500 micrograms in 2 mL. Digoxin 150 micrograms is prescribed.

8   Stock Calciparine contains 25 000 units in 1 mL. 15 000 units of Calciparine is prescribed.

9   Penicillin 450 mg at 2000 hrs is prescribed. Stock ampoules contain 600 mg in 5 mL.

Check your answers on p 158

Exercise 3E *Calculate the volume of stock solution to be drawn up for injection.*

Give answers greater than 1 mL correct to one decimal place and answers less than 1 mL correct to two decimal places. If the next decimal place is 5 or more, add one to the previous digit.

1 *Prescribed:* erythromycin 200 mg
  Stock: 300 mg in 10 mL

2 *Prescribed:* morphine 20 mg
  Stock: 15 mg in 1 mL

3 *Prescribed:* atropine 0.5 mg
  Stock: 0.6 mg in 1 mL

4 *Prescribed:* atropine 800 micrograms
  Stock: 1.2 mg in 1 mL

5 *Prescribed:* naloxone 0.35 mg
  Stock: 0.4 mg/mL

6 *Prescribed:* capreomycin 850 mg
  Stock: 2 g per mL

7 *Prescribed:* metoclopramide 7 mg
  Stock: 10 mg/2 mL

8 *Prescribed:* heparin 1750 units
  Stock: 1000 units per mL

9 *Prescribed:* buscopan 0.25 mg
  Stock: 0.4 mg/2 mL

If you are having difficulty with rounding off decimal answers, then refer to Review exercise 1K in Chapter 1.

Check your answers on p 159

Exercise 3F *Calculate the volume of stock required. Give answers greater than 1 mL correct to one decimal place and answers less than 1 mL correct to two decimal places.*

	Prescribed	Dosage	Stock ampoule
1	Morphine	12 mg	15 mg/mL
2	Calciparine	7000 units	25 000 units in 1 mL
3	Benzylpenicillin	1500 mg	1.2 g in 10 mL
4	Heparin	3000 units	5000 units per mL
5	Phenobarbitone	70 mg	200 mg/mL
6	Pethidine	80 mg	100 mg in 2 mL
7	Buscopan	0.24 mg	0.4 mg/2 mL
8	Digoxin	200 micrograms	500 micrograms in 2 mL
9	Furosemide (frusemide)	150 mg	250 mg in 5 mL
10	Ondansetron	5 mg	4 mg in 2 mL
11	Capreomycin	800 mg	1 g in 5 mL
12	Tramadol	120 mg	100 mg in 2 mL
13	Gentamicin	70 mg	80 mg in 2 mL
14	Vancomycin	750 mg	1 g in 5 mL
15	Morphine	7.5 mg	10 mg in 1 mL
16	Ceftriaxone	1250 mg	1 g/3 mL
17	Buscopan	25 mg	20 mg in 1 mL
18	Dexamethasone	3 mg	4 mg/mL
19	Vancomycin	1.2 g	1000 mg/5 mL
20	Naloxone	0.5 mg	0.4 mg/mL

Check your answers on p 159

CALCULATIONS FOR INJECTION INVOLVING PRESCRIPTIONS AND MEDICATION LABELS

Exercise 3G *Read each prescription and medication label carefully. Each medication label refers to the stock available in the ward. Calculate the volume to be drawn up in the syringe.*

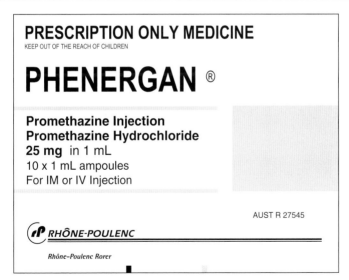

1

Regular medicines

Year 20 16		Date and month ⟶	4/5								
PRESCRIBER MUST ENTER administration times ⟶											

Date 4/5	Medicine (print generic name) PROMETHAZINE	Tick if slow release	0800 h.						Continue on discharge? Yes / No
Route IM	Dose 20 mg	Frequency and NOW enter times BD	1200 ½n						Dispense? Yes / No days Qty:
Indication URTICARIA		Pharmacy							Duration: Date:
Prescriber signature ৸	Print your name Li	Contact 712							

PRESCRIPTION ONLY MEDICINE
KEEP OUT OF THE REACH OF CHILDREN

PHENERGAN ®

Promethazine Injection
Promethazine Hydrochloride
25 mg in 1 mL
10 x 1 mL ampoules
For IM or IV Injection

AUST R 27545

℗ RHÔNE-POULENC

Rhône–Poulenc Rorer

Check your answers on p 159

2

Regular medicines

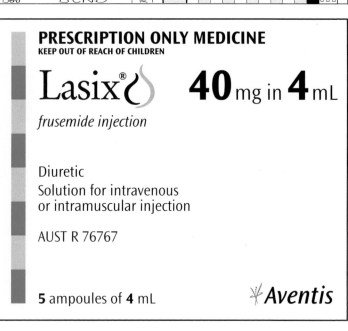

Year 20 16			Date and month ➝	14/11	15/11	16/11							
PRESCRIBER MUST ENTER administration times ➤													

Date 14/11	Medicine (print generic name) FRUSEMIDE	Tick if slow release	0800 7.9 PR								Continue on discharge? Yes / No
Route IV	Dose 60mg	Frequency and NOW enter times MANE ➝									Dispense? Yes / No
Indication HEART FAILURE		Pharmacy									days Qty:
Prescriber signature Bend	Print your name BEND	Contact 124									Duration: Date:

PRESCRIPTION ONLY MEDICINE
KEEP OUT OF REACH OF CHILDREN

Lasix® ♀   **40** mg in **4** mL

frusemide injection

Diuretic
Solution for intravenous
or intramuscular injection

AUST R 76767

5 ampoules of **4** mL   ⚕*Aventis*

Check your answers on p 159

3

Regular medicines

Year 20 _16_		Date and month ⟶	11/12												Continue on discharge? Yes / No	Dispense? Yes / No		Date:

First prescriber to print patient name
and check label correct:

Date _11/12_	Medicine (print generic name) PROMETHAZINE		Tick if slow release	Date 11/12				
Route M	Dose Hourly frequency _12.5 mg_	Max PRN dose/24 hrs 3		Time 0630				
		PRN						
Indication URTICARIA	Pharmacy			Dose 12.5				
				Route IM				
Prescriber signature PK	Print your name KORT	Contact 156		Sign 2				

PRESCRIPTION ONLY MEDICINE
KEEP OUT OF THE REACH OF CHILDREN

PHENERGAN ®

Promethazine Injection
Promethazine Hydrochloride
25 mg in 1 mL
10 x 1 mL ampoules
For IM or IV Injection

AUST R 27545

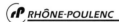 **RHÔNE-POULENC**

Rhône–Poulenc Rorer

4

Regular medicines

Year 20 16			Date and month →	³/₁₀	⁴/₁₀	⁵/₁₀								
PRESCRIBER MUST ENTER administration times														
Date 3/10	Medicine (print generic name) FRUSEMIDE		Tick if slow release											
Route IV	Dose 35 mg	Frequency and NOW enter times BD →		0800	⁊⁊	⅃ₒ								
Indication O EDEMA		Pharmacy		1200	⁊⁊	⅃⁊								
Prescriber signature Kodgi	Print your name KODGI		Contact 891											

PRESCRIPTION ONLY MEDICINE
KEEP OUT OF REACH OF CHILDREN

Lasix®

frusemide injection

20 mg in **2** mL

Diuretic

Solution for intravenous
or intramuscular injection

AUST R 12404

5 ampoules of **2** mL   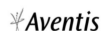 *Aventis*

Check your answers on p 159

MEASURING VOLUMES FOR INJECTION USING SYRINGES

Exercise 3H *The drawings represent syringes (needles not shown)*

1 For this set of 1 mL syringes, write down the volume (mL) of solution
   a between adjacent graduations
   b indicated by arrows A, B, C and D.

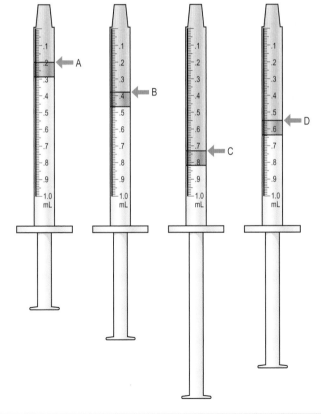

Check your answers on p 159

2   For this set of three syringes, write down the volume (mL) of solution
    a between adjacent graduations
    b indicated by arrows A, B and C.

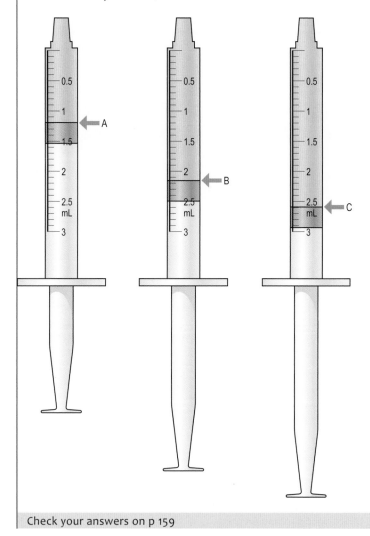

Check your answers on p 159

3 For these syringes, write down the volume (mL) of solution
  a between adjacent graduations
  b indicated by arrows A, B and C.

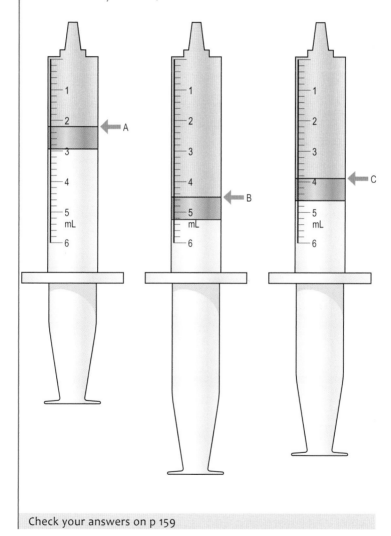

Check your answers on p 159

4 For these 10 mL syringes, write down the volume (mL) of solution
  a between adjacent graduations
  b indicated by arrows A, B and C.

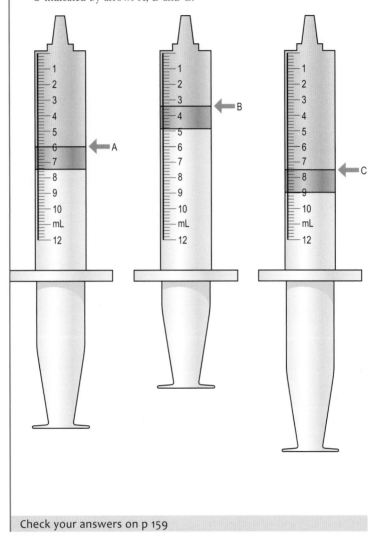

Dosages of Medications for Injection

5   These syringes are graduated in *units*, especially for *insulin* injections.
    Write down the number of units of solution
    a between adjacent graduations
    b indicated by arrows A, B, C and D.

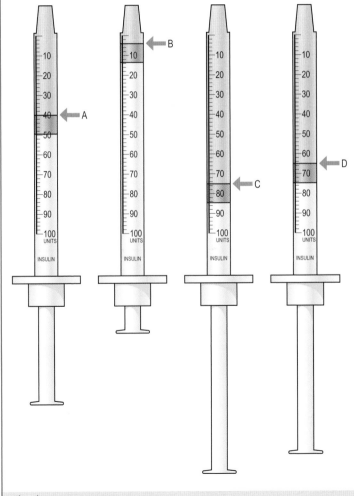

Check your answers on p 159

Nursing Calculations

6 For these 50 unit syringes, identify the number of units of solution
   a between adjacent graduations
   b indicated by arrows A, B, C and D.

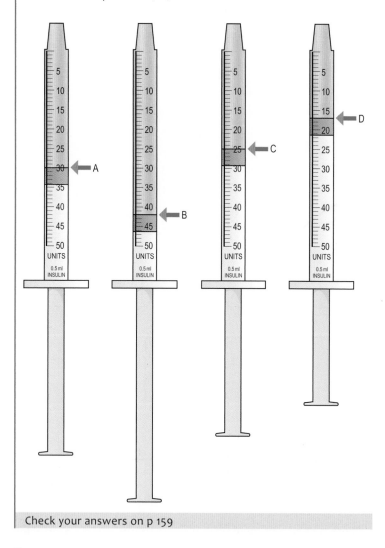

Check your answers on p 159

7 For these 50 unit syringes, note carefully the number of units of
   solution
   a between adjacent graduations
   b indicated by arrows A, B, C and D.

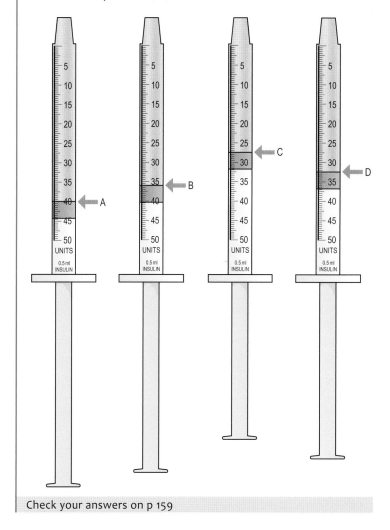

Check your answers on p 159

Nursing Calculations

CHAPTER 3 REVISION

1   Phenobarbitone 60 mg is to be given at 1600 hrs by IM injection. Stock ampoules contain 200 mg per mL. Is the volume of stock required equal to 1 mL, less than 1 mL, or more than 1 mL?

2   Pethidine 70 mg stat is to be given IM. Calculate the volume of stock required if ampoules contain pethidine 100 mg in 2 mL.

3   Heparin 12 000 units subcut at 0800 hrs is prescribed. Stock ampoules contain 25 000 units/5 mL. What volume should be drawn up?

4   A patient is prescribed benzylpenicillin 900 mg. On hand is benzylpenicillin 600 mg in 5 mL (once diluted). Calculate the volume to be drawn up for injection.

5   Digoxin ampoules on hand contain 500 micrograms in 2 mL. What volume is needed for an injection of 275 micrograms?

6   A patient is prescribed tramadol hydrochloride 75 mg IM at 1700 hrs. Ampoules contain tramadol hydrochloride 100 mg in 2 mL. Calculate the volume required for injection.

7   A patient is prescribed vancomycin 900 mg IV. Calculate the amount of stock solution required if stock on hand contains 1 g per 10 mL.

8   Buscopan 0.18 mg is prescribed. Stock ampoules contain 0.4 mg/2 mL. Calculate the volume to be drawn up for injection.

9   A patient is to be given an injection of erythromycin 190 mg at 1900 hrs. Stock ampoules contain 300 mg/10 mL. Calculate the required volume.

10   How much morphine must be drawn up for a 10 mg dose if a stock ampoule contains 15 mg in 1 mL?

Check your answers on p 160

Intravenous infusion 4

This chapter deals with the arithmetic of flow rates and drip rates for intravenous (IV) infusion.

The fluid being infused passes from a flask (or similar container) into a giving set (administration set), which has a drip chamber. The giving set may be free-hanging or attached to a volumetric infusion pump.

If the giving set is free-hanging, the nurse needs to calculate the drops per minute to be infused. The nurse can then manipulate the roller clamp on the giving set to ensure the drip rate is correct.

By contrast, if the giving set is connected to an infusion pump, then the nurse needs only to calculate the number of millilitres per hour to be infused and set the pump accordingly.

> There may be a burette between the flask and the giving set. The use of a burette will depend on institution policy and the type of infusion.

There are two *main* types of giving sets in general use – these break down fluid into a *drop factor* of either 20 or 60 drops per mL. A drip chamber that delivers 60 drops per mL (or has a *drop factor* of 60 drops/mL) is also known as a *microdrip*. Another giving set with a drop factor of 15 drops/mL is used occasionally.

Skills covered in this chapter include:

- calculating the volume of fluid delivered to a patient over a given time
- infusion pump settings
- rates of flow in mL/hr
- rates of flow in drops/min.

24-hour time will be used in some exercises.

Important: If in **any** doubt about the answer to a calculation, then ask a supervisor to check your work.

Refer to prelim page ix for explanations of abbreviations.

CALCULATING VOLUME OF AN INFUSION

Example *A patient is receiving 5% dextrose by IV infusion. The drip rate is set to deliver 45 mL per hour. Calculate how much fluid the patient will receive in each case.*

How much fluid will the patient receive

a over 2 hrs   b over 3 hrs   c over 7 hrs?

$$\text{Volume (mL)} = \text{Rate (mL/hr)} \times \text{Time (hr)}$$

a 45 mL/hr $\times$ 2 hr = 90 mL
b 45 mL/hr $\times$ 3 hr = 135 mL
c 45 mL/hr $\times$ 7 hr = 315 mL

CALCULATING TIME FOR AN INFUSION

Example *A teenager is to receive 750 mL of Hartmann's solution. An infusion pump is set at 60 mL/hr. How long will it take to give the solution?*

$$\text{Time (hr)} = \frac{\text{Volume (mL)}}{\text{Rate (mL/hr)}}$$

$$= \frac{750 \text{ mL}}{60 \text{ mL/hr}}$$

$$= 12\tfrac{1}{2} \text{ hours or } 12 \text{ hr } 30 \text{ min}$$

$$\text{Simplifying}: \frac{750}{60} = \frac{75}{6} = \frac{25}{2} = 12\tfrac{1}{2}$$

Exercise 4A

1 An intravenous line has been inserted in a patient. Fluid is being delivered at a rate of 42 mL/hr. How much fluid will the patient receive over **a** 2 hrs **b** 8 hrs **c** 12 hrs?

2 A male patient is receiving Hartmann's solution at a rate of 125 mL/hr. How much solution will he receive over **a** 3 hrs **b** 5 hrs **c** 12 hrs?

3 A girl is to be given 5% dextrose via an infusion pump. If the pump is set at 60 mL/hr, how much 5% dextrose will she receive in **a** $1\frac{1}{2}$ hrs **b** $2\frac{1}{2}$ hrs **c** 12 hrs?

4 A female patient is to receive 500 mL of 0.9% sodium chloride. The drip rate is adjusted to deliver 25 mL/hr. How long will the fluid last?

5 A young man is to be given one litre of 4% dextrose and $\frac{1}{5}$ normal saline. The infusion pump is set at a rate of 80 mL/hr. What time will it take to give the litre of solution?

6 Half a litre of normal saline with 2 g potassium chloride is to be given to a patient IV. How long will this take if the infusion pump is set at 75 mL/hr?

7 A patient is to receive 100 mL of 0.9% sodium chloride IV. If the infusion pump is set to deliver 150 mL/hr, how long will the infusion take?

Check your answers on p 161

CALCULATING RATES OF FLOW IN MILLILITRES PER HOUR (mL/hr) *GIVEN THE TIME IN HOURS*

In order to do this type of calculation, you will need to remember this formula:

$$\text{Rate (mL/hr)} = \frac{\text{Volume (mL)}}{\text{Time (hr)}}$$

Note: The volume must be in millilitres (mL).

Example *A patient is to receive half a litre of fluid IV over 6 hours using an infusion pump. At how many millilitres per hour should the pump be set?*

The pump does not have a decimal setting, so calculate the answer to the nearest whole number.

Half a litre = 500 mL

$$\text{Rate (mL/hr)} = \frac{\text{Volume (mL)}}{\text{Time (hr)}}$$

$$= \frac{500 \text{ mL}}{6 \text{ hr}}$$

$$= \frac{250}{3} \text{ mL/hr}$$

$$\Rightarrow 83 \text{ mL/hr (to nearest whole number)}$$

$$3)\overline{25^10.^10}$$
$$83.\underline{3}$$

Exercise 4B *Calculate the required flow rate of a volumetric infusion pump for each of the following infusions.*

Give answers in mL/hr to the nearest whole number.

1   One litre of normal saline is to be administered over 8 hours.

2   A patient is to receive 500 mL of 5% dextrose over 12 hours.

3   500 mL of Hartmann's solution is to be given to a teenager over 7 hours.

4   Over the next 15 hours, a female patient is to receive 2 L of 4% dextrose and $\frac{1}{5}$ normal saline.

5   A teenager is to receive one litre of 0.9% sodium chloride over 6 hours.

6   A woman is to be given 500 mL of 5% dextrose over 8 hours.

7   Over a period of 16 hours, a patient is to receive one litre of 4% dextrose and 0.18% sodium chloride.

8   A patient is to be given one litre of normal saline over 24 hours.

9   Over the next 9 hours, a patient is to receive half a litre of 4% dextrose and $\frac{1}{5}$ normal saline. At what flow rate should the volumetric infusion pump be set?

10 One litre of Hartmann's solution is to be given over 12 hours. Calculate the required flow rate for the volumetric infusion pump.

Check your answers on p 161

CALCULATING RATES OF FLOW IN MILLILITRES PER HOUR (mL/hr) *GIVEN THE TIME IN MINUTES*

In order to do this type of calculation, you will need to remember the final formula below:

$$60 \text{ minutes} = 1 \text{ hour}$$

$$60 \text{ min} = 1 \text{ hr}$$

$$\text{Rate (mL/min)} = \frac{\text{Volume (mL)}}{\text{Time (min)}}$$

$$\text{Rate (mL/hr)} = \text{Rate (mL/min)} \times 60$$

$$\therefore \text{Rate (mL/hr)} = \frac{\text{Volume (mL)} \times 60}{\text{Time (min)}}$$

Note:

The volume must be in millilitres (mL).

The time must be in minutes (min).

Example *75 mL of fluid in a burette needs to be infused over 20 minutes. Calculate the flow rate required in mL/hr.*

$$\text{Rate (mL/hr)} = \frac{\text{Volume (mL)} \times 60}{\text{Time (min)}}$$

$$= \frac{75 \text{ mL} \times 60}{20 \text{ min}}$$

$$= 225 \text{ mL/hr}$$

Exercise 4C *Each of the following medications has been added to a burette. Calculate the required pump setting in mL/hr for the given infusion time. Give each answer to the nearest whole number.*

	Medication	Infusion time
1	40 mL of fluid containing 600 mg of penicillin	20 minutes
2	120 mL of fluid containing 500 mg of vancomycin	50 minutes
3	100 mL of fluid containing 1 g of flucloxacillin	30 minutes
4	50 mL of fluid containing 0.5 g of potassium chloride	half an hour
5	60 mL of fluid containing 75 mg of ranitidine	35 minutes
6	80 mL of fluid containing 80 mg of gentamicin	45 minutes
7	75 mL of fluid containing 75 mg of gentamicin	40 minutes
8	70 mL of fluid containing 1.2 g of penicillin	25 minutes
9	80 mL of fluid containing 750 mg of flucloxacillin	half an hour
10	100 mL of fluid containing metronidazole 500 mg	half an hour

Check your answers on p 161

CALCULATING RATES OF FLOW IN DROPS PER MINUTE (DROPS/MIN)

When a giving set is free-hanging (no pump is being used), the nurse needs to calculate the flow rate in drops/min. This is so that the nurse can set the drip rate accurately by manipulating the roller clamp while observing the drip chamber on the giving set.

Note: Before commencing the calculation always make sure that you know the *drop factor* for the drip chamber of that giving set. The *drop factor* could be 20 drops/mL (delivers fluid at 20 drops per mL), 60 drops/mL (delivers fluid at 60 drops per mL) or 15 drops/mL (delivers fluid at 15 drops per mL).

In order to do this type of calculation, you will need to remember these formulae:

If the time is given in *minutes* use:

$$\text{Rate (drops/min)} = \frac{\text{Volume (mL)} \times \text{Drop factor (drops/mL)}}{\text{Time (minutes)}}$$

If the time is given in *hours* use:

$$\text{Rate (drops/min)} = \frac{\text{Volume (mL)} \times \text{Drop factor (drops/mL)}}{\text{Time (hours)} \times 60}$$

Note: The volume must be in millilitres (mL).

Note: Calculating flow rates in drops/min does not apply when an infusion is being delivered via a volumetric pump, as the pump setting regulates the drops.

Example *A patient is prescribed half a litre of 5% dextrose over 4 hours. The drip chamber in the administration set delivers 20 drops/mL. Calculate the required drip rate in drops/min.*

Give the answer to the nearest whole number.

Note: Half a litre = 500 mL. Time is given in hours.

$$\text{Rate (drops/min)} = \frac{\text{Volume (mL)} \times \text{Drop factor (drops/mL)}}{\text{Time (hours)} \times 60}$$

$$= \frac{500\,\text{mL} \times 20\,\text{drops/mL}}{4\,\text{hr} \times 60}$$

$$= \frac{500 \times 20\,\text{drops}}{4 \times 60\,\text{min}}$$

$$= \frac{500}{4} \times \frac{1}{3}\,\text{drops/min} \left[\text{since}\,\frac{20}{60} = \frac{1}{3} \right]$$

$$= \frac{125}{3}\,\text{drops/min} \left[\text{since}\,\frac{500}{4} = 125 \right] \qquad \frac{41.\textcircled{6}}{3)\,125.^{2}0}$$

$$\Rightarrow 42\,\text{drops/min}$$

Note: In this example the nurse is required to adjust the roller clamp to set the drip rate accurately (drops/min).

Nursing Calculations

Exercise 4D *Calculate the required drip rate in drops per minute.*

Give each answer to the nearest whole number.

1 750 mL of 5% dextrose is to be given over 5 hours. The IV set delivers 20 drops per millilitre.

2 An infant is prescribed 150 mL of Hartmann's solution to run over 6 hours. The microdrip delivers 60 drops per millilitre.

3 A teenager is to receive 500 mL of 5% dextrose over 8 hours. The IV set emits 20 drops/mL.

4 0.5 litre of dextrose 4% and $\frac{1}{5}$ normal saline is to run over 12 hours. The administration set delivers 20 drops/mL.

5 750 mL of normal saline is to be given to a patient over 9 hours using a giving set which emits 20 drops/mL.

6 An adult male is to be given half a litre of 0.9% sodium chloride over 5 hours using an IV set which gives 20 drops per millilitre.

7 A female patient is to receive $1\frac{1}{2}$ litres of fluid over 10 hours. The giving set delivers 20 drops/mL.

8 A patient is to have the remaining 300 mL of 5% dextrose run through in 50 minutes. The administration set gives 20 drops/mL.

9 400 mL of normal saline is to be infused over 10 hours using a microdrop giving set. The set delivers 60 drops/mL.

10 A child is prescribed 24 mL/hr of 0.9% sodium chloride. The micro-drop delivers 60 drops/mL.

11 An antibiotic has been added to the burette. The burette then contains 120 mL of fluid that needs to be delivered in 30 minutes. The administration set gives 20 drops/mL.

12 A male patient is to have the remaining 50 mL of 5% dextrose infused in 45 minutes. The administration set gives 20 drops/mL.

Check your answers on p 162

CALCULATING RATES OF FLOW FOR BLOOD TRANSFUSIONS (DROPS/MIN)

Example *One unit of packed cells is prescribed to be infused over 2 hours. The volume of the unit of packed cells is 250 mL. The IV set emits 20 drops/mL. Calculate the drip rate in drops/min.*

Give the answer to the nearest whole number.

Note: Time is given in hours.

$$\text{Rate (drops/min)} = \frac{\text{Volume (mL)} \times \text{Drop factor (drops/mL)}}{\text{Time (hours)} \times 60}$$

$$= \frac{250 \, \text{mL} \times 20 \, \text{drops/mL}}{2 \, \text{hr} \times 60}$$

$$= \frac{250 \times 20 \, \text{drops}}{2 \times 60 \, \text{min}}$$

$$= \frac{250}{2} \times \frac{1}{3} \, \text{drops/min} \left[\text{since} \frac{20}{60} = \frac{1}{3} \right]$$

$$= \frac{125}{3} \, \text{drops/min}$$

$$\Rightarrow 42 \, \text{drops/min}$$

$$3 \overline{)\, 125.^{2}0}$$
$$\underline{41.\text{⑥}}$$

Note: In this example the nurse is required to adjust the roller clamp to set the drip rate accurately (drops/min).

Exercise 4E *Calculate the drip rate in drops per minute for each of the following blood transfusions.*

Give each answer to the nearest whole number.

1   An anaemic patient is prescribed 1 unit of packed cells over 4 hours. The unit of packed cells holds 250 mL. The IV set delivers 20 drops per mL.

2   A post-operative adult male is to be given 1 unit of autologous blood in 4 hours. The unit of autologous blood has a volume of 500 mL. The giving set emits 20 drops/mL.

3   During a transfusion, the doctor prescribes the remaining half unit of packed cells to be administered over one hour. A full unit of packed cells is 250 mL. The IV giving set delivers 20 drops per mL.

4   300 mL of autologous blood is to be transfused over 2 hours using an administration set which gives 20 drops per mL.

5   One unit of packed red cells is to be run over 3 hours. The unit of packed cells contains 350 mL. An IV set which emits 15 drops/mL is to be used.

6   A patient is to be given 1 unit of autologous blood over 3 hours using a giving set which delivers 15 drops/mL. The unit of blood contains 480 mL.

7   An administration set which emits 15 drops/mL is to be used to give a 480 mL unit of autologous blood over $3\frac{1}{2}$ hours.

8   A 350 mL unit of packed cells is to be run over $2\frac{1}{2}$ hours using an IV giving set which delivers 15 drops/mL.

Check your answers on p 162

CALCULATING FINISHING TIMES OF INTRAVENOUS INFUSIONS

Example A *A patient is ordered 1 litre of normal saline to be run over $12\frac{1}{2}$ hours. If the infusion begins at 0800 hours Monday, calculate the finishing time.*

0800 hours Monday + 12 hr 30 min = 2030 hours Monday

Example B *A patient is to be given 1 litre of 5% dextrose over 18 hours, starting at 0930 hours Wednesday. Calculate the finishing time.*

0930 hours Wednesday + 18 hr 00 min = 2730 hours

But there are only 24 hours in a day

2730 hrs – 2400 hrs = 0330 hours Thursday

Exercise 4F *Calculate the finishing time of each infusion.*

Give each answer in 24-hour time and include the day.

1   *Ordered:* 500 mL normal saline
    Running time: 6 hr 30 min
    Starting time: 0900 Tuesday

2   *Ordered:* 1 litre dextrose 4% and $\frac{1}{5}$ normal saline
    Running time: 13 hours
    Starting time: Noon Sunday

3   *Ordered:* 1 litre of Hartmann's solution
    Running time: 14 hours
    Starting time: 0730 Friday

4   *Ordered:* Half a litre of dextrose 5%
    Running time: $10\frac{1}{2}$ hours
    Starting time: 1715 Thursday

5   *Ordered:* 1.2 L of 0.9% sodium chloride
    Running time: $13\frac{1}{2}$ hours
    Starting time: 1030 Monday

6   *Ordered:* 1.25 L of 4% dextrose and 0.18% sodium chloride
    Running time: 21 hours
    Starting time: 0900 Saturday

7   *Ordered:* One litre of Hartmann's solution
    Running time: $11\frac{1}{2}$ hours
    Starting time: 1300 Wednesday

Check your answers on p 162

CALCULATING RUNNING TIMES AND FINISHING TIMES OF INTRAVENOUS INFUSIONS

In order to do this type of calculation, you will need to remember the formulae used in the next two examples.

Example A *At 0730 hours, a 500 mL flask of 0.9% sodium chloride is set up to run at 80 mL/hr. At what time would the flask have to be replaced?*

$$\text{Running time (hours)} = \frac{\text{Volume (mL)}}{\text{Rate (mL/hr)}}$$

$$= \frac{500 \text{ mL}}{80 \text{ mL/hr}}$$

$$= 6\frac{1}{4} \text{ hr or 6 hr 15 min}$$

$\therefore$ Finishing time $= 0730 \text{ hr} + 6 \text{ hr } 15 \text{ min} = 1345 \text{ hours}$

Example B *At 0600 hours, a one litre flask of normal saline is set up to run through an infusion pump at 70 mL/hr. After 8 hours, the flow rate prescribed is to be increased to 80 mL/hr. By what time would the flask have to be replaced?*

    i   Volume (mL) = Rate (mL/hr) $\times$ Time (hr)

           = 70 mL/hr $\times$ 8 hr = 560 mL

    ii   One litre = 1000 mL

    $\therefore$ Volume remaining = 1000 mL − 560 mL = 440 mL

    iii   Running time (hours) $= \dfrac{\text{Volume (mL)}}{\text{Rate (mL/hr)}}$

$$= \frac{440 \text{ mL}}{80 \text{ mL/hr}}$$

$$= 5\frac{1}{2} \text{ hr or 5 hr 30 min}$$

    iv   Total running time = 8 hr + $5\frac{1}{2}$ hr = $13\frac{1}{2}$ hr or 13 hr 30 min

    v $\therefore$ Finishing time = 0600 hr + 13 hr 30 min = 1930 hours

Nursing Calculations

Exercise 4G

1   A patient has *two* intravenous lines. One line is being infused at 45 mL/ hr; the other at 30 mL/hr. What volume of fluid would this patient receive in a 24-hour period?

2   At 0800 hours, one litre of 4% dextrose and 0.18% sodium chloride is set up to run at 75 mL/hr. At what time would the flask be finished?

3   At 2100 hours on a Monday, one litre of 5% dextrose is set up to run at 50 mL/hr. When will the flask be finished?

4   One litre of Hartmann's solution is to be given IV. For the first 6 hours the solution is delivered at 85 mL/hr, then the rate is prescribed to be reduced to 70 mL/hr. Find the total time taken to give the full volume.

5   A patient is to receive half a litre of 5% dextrose IV. A flask is set up at 0800 hours running at 60 mL/hr. After 5 hours the rate is prescribed to be increased to 80 mL/hr. At what time will the IV be completed?

6   At 0430 hours, an infusion pump is set to deliver 1.5 L of fluid at a rate of 90 mL/hr. After 10 hours the pump is reset to 75 mL/hr. Calculate the finishing time.

7   A one litre IV flask of 0.9% sodium chloride has been infused for 6 hours at a rate of 75 mL/hr. The doctor prescribes the remaining volume to be run through in the next 5 hours. Calculate the new flow rate.

8   A patient is to receive one litre of 4% dextrose and 0.18% sodium chloride. For the first $3\frac{1}{2}$ hours the fluid is delivered at 160 mL/hr. A specialist then prescribes that the rate be slowed so that the remaining fluid will run over the next 8 hours. Calculate the required flow rate.

Check your answers on p 162

CALCULATING STOCK CONCENTRATION AND ADMINISTRATION OF DOSAGES

In order to do this type of calculation, you will need to remember the following four formulae:

1   To calculate the concentration of a stock solution use:

$$\text{Concentration of stock (mg/mL)} = \frac{\text{Stock strength (mg)}}{\text{Volume of stock solution (mL)}}$$

2   To calculate the amount of medication contained in a given volume use:

$$\text{Dosage (mg)} = \text{Volume (mL)} \times \text{Concentration of stock (mg/mL)}$$

3   To calculate the amount of medication received per hour use:

$$\text{Hourly dosage (mg/hr)} = \text{Rate (mL/hr)} \times \text{Concentration of stock (mg/mL)}$$

4   To calculate the rate in millilitres per hour use:

$$\text{Rate (mL/hr)} = \frac{\text{Hourly dosage (mg/hr)}}{\text{Concentration of stock (mg/mL)}}$$

Nursing Calculations

Example A *A young post-operative patient's IV analgesic prescription is for pethidine 300 mg in 500 mL of normal saline. The solution is prescribed to run between 10 and 40 mL/hr, depending on the nurse's assessment of pain.*

a   **Calculate the concentration of the pethidine/saline solution.**
b   **How many milligrams of pethidine will the patient receive each hour if the infusion is run at 25 mL/hr?**
c   **At what rate (in mL/hr) should the nurse set the pump to administer the pethidine at 8 mg/hr? Give answer to nearest whole number.**

a   Concentration $= \dfrac{300 \text{ mg}}{500 \text{ mL}} = \dfrac{3}{5}$ mg/mL or 0.6 mg/mL

b   Hourly dosage $= 25$ mL/hr $\times 0.6$ mg/mL $= 15$ mg/hr

c   Rate $= \dfrac{8 \text{ mg/hr}}{0.6 \text{ mg/mL}} = \dfrac{80}{6}$ mL/hr $= 13.3 \Rightarrow 13$ m

$$6 \overline{)\, 8^2 0.^2 0}$$
$$\frac{\quad\quad}{13.\textcircled{3}}$$

Example B *A post-operative female patient has a patient-controlled analgesia (PCA) infusion. The flask contains morphine 50 mg in 100 mL of normal saline. The PCA has been set, as per doctor's prescription, so that when the patient presses the button she receives a bolus dose of 1 mL.*

a   **Calculate the concentration of the morphine/saline solution.**
b   **How much morphine does the bolus dose contain?**

a   Concentration $= \dfrac{50 \text{ mg}}{100 \text{ mL}} = \dfrac{1}{2}$ mg/mL $= 0.5$ mg/mL

b   Dosage (mg) = Volume (mL)×Concentration of stock (mg/mL)

$\therefore$ Dosage $= 1$ mL$\times 0.5$ mg/mL $= 0.5$ mg

Exercise 4H

1 A young post-operative patient is prescribed pethidine 350 mg in 500 mL of normal saline. The solution is prescribed to infuse between 10 and 40 mL/hr, depending on the nurse's assessment of pain.

   a What is the concentration (mg/mL) of the pethidine/saline solution?

   b How many milligrams of pethidine will the patient receive hourly if the infusion is run at:

     i   10 mL/hr   ii   15 mL/hr

     iii 25 mL/hr   iv 40 mL/hr?

   c At what rate (mL/hr) should the pump be set to deliver the pethidine at:

     i   9 mg/hr   ii   12 mg/hr

     iii 20 mg/hr   iv 25 mg/hr?

   [Give each answer to nearest whole number.]

2 An adult male patient is prescribed morphine 50 mg in 500 mL of normal saline. The solution is to be infused at 10–40 mL/hr using a volumetric infusion pump.

   a Calculate the concentration (mg/mL) of the morphine/saline solution.

   b How many milligrams of morphine will the patient receive per hour if the pump is set at:

     i   10 mL/hr   ii   15 mL/hr

     iii 20 mL/hr   iv 40 mL/hr?

   c At what rate (mL/hr) should the pump be set to deliver the morphine at:

     i   1.5 mg/hr   ii   2.5 mg/hr

     iii 3 mg/hr   iv 3.5 mg/hr?

3 A post-operative patient has a patient-controlled analgesia (PCA) infusion running via a syringe pump. The syringe contains fentanyl 300 micrograms in 30 mL of 0.9% sodium chloride. The PCA has been set, in accordance with doctor's prescription, so that when the button is pressed the patient receives a bolus dose of 1 mL.

   a What is the concentration (microgram/mL) of the solution in the syringe?

   b How much fentanyl is in each bolus dose?

   c If the patient has six bolus doses within an hour, how much fentanyl has the patient received in that hour?

Check your answers on p 163

CALCULATING KILOJOULES OF ENERGY

Calculating the number of kilojoules a patient receives from an intravenous infusion is not something that a nurse does on a regular basis. However, in certain patient situations it is beneficial to be aware of the number of kilojoules the patient is receiving from the infusion.

Note: Dextrose and glucose are carbohydrates. The given percentage of dextrose (or glucose) is equal to the number of grams of dextrose (or glucose) per 100 mL of solution.
For example:

5% dextrose = 5 g of dextrose per 100 mL of solution

10% dextrose = 10 g of dextrose per 100 mL of solution

25% dextrose = 25 g of dextrose per 100 mL of solution

50% dextrose = 50 g of dextrose per 100 mL of solution

Example *One gram of dextrose provides 16 kilojoules of energy. How many kilojoules does a patient receive from an infusion of $1\frac{1}{2}$ litres of 10% dextrose?*

$$10\% \text{ dextrose} = 10 \text{ g of dextrose per } 100 \text{ mL of solution}$$
$$= \frac{10 \text{ g}}{100 \text{ mL}}$$
$$1\frac{1}{2} \text{ litres} = 1500 \text{ mL}$$

Weight of dextrose (g) = Volume of infusion (mL)
$$\times \text{ strength of solution (g/100 mL)}$$
$$= 1500 \text{ mL} \times \frac{10 \text{ g}}{100 \text{ mL}}$$
$$= \frac{1500 \text{ mL}}{1} \times \frac{10 \text{ g}}{100 \text{ mL}}$$
$$= 15 \times 10 \text{ g} \qquad (1500 \text{ mL} \div 100 \text{ mL} = 15)$$
$$= 150 \text{ g}$$

Energy supplied $= 150 \text{ g} \times 16 \text{ kJ/g}$
$$= 2400 \text{ kJ}$$

Exercise 4I *One gram of carbohydrate provides 16 kilojoules of energy. Dextrose and glucose are carbohydrates. Calculate how many kilojoules will be received by a patient in each of the following infusions.*

1   1 L of 5% dextrose

2   $2\frac{1}{2}$ L of 5% dextrose

3   1 L of 10% dextrose

4   500 mL of 25% dextrose

5   2 L of normal saline
    [Normal saline is a 0.9% solution of salt in water.]

6   750 mL of 4% dextrose and $\frac{1}{5}$ normal saline

7   $1\frac{1}{2}$ L of Hartmann's solution
    [Hartmann's solution contains sodium lactate, sodium chloride, potassium chloride and calcium chloride.]

8   A patient with diabetes is found unconscious and presumed to be hypoglycaemic. 50 mL of 50% glucose is given to the patient. How many kilojoules of energy are administered in the 50 mL dose?

Check your answers on p 163

CHAPTER 4 REVISION

1   A male patient is receiving 5% dextrose at a rate of 55 mL/hr. How much fluid will he receive in **a** 2 hr, **b** 5 hr, **c** 11 hr?

2   A patient is to receive one litre of Hartmann's solution. If an infusion pump is set at 120 mL/hr, how long will the pump take to give the solution?

3   1.5 L of 4% dextrose and 0.18% sodium chloride over 20 hr is prescribed for a patient. Calculate the required flow rate setting for a volumetric infusion pump.

4   An infusion pump is to be used to administer one litre of fluid over 11 hours. At what flow rate should the pump be set?

5   100 mL of fluid containing vancomycin 400 mg has been added to a burette. The infusion is to be given over 45 minutes. Calculate the required pump setting in mL/hr, to the nearest whole number.

6   600 mL of normal saline is to be infused over 12 hours using a microdrop giving set. The set delivers 60 drops per millilitre. Calculate the required drip rate in drops per minute.

7   One unit of packed cells is to be given to a patient over 3 hours. The giving set delivers 20 drops/mL. Calculate the drip rate in drops/min if one unit of packed cells contains 250 mL. Give the answer to the nearest whole number.

8   A patient is to be given $1\frac{1}{2}$ litres of fluid over 10 hours. The giving set emits 20 drops/mL. Calculate the required drip rate in drops/min.

9   A female patient is to receive one litre of Hartmann's solution over 12 hours. Calculate the drip rate if the administration set gives 15 drops/mL.

10 A patient is receiving fluid from *two* IV lines. One line is running at 65 mL/hr; the other at 70 mL/hr. What volume of fluid would the patient receive IV over 12 hours?

11 At 0700 hours, half a litre of 5% dextrose is set up to run at 40 mL/hr. At what time will the flask be finished?

12 A litre of 5% dextrose is to be given IV. The solution is to run at 75 mL/hr for the first 6 hours, then the rate is to be reduced to 50 mL/hr. Calculate the *total* time required to give the full volume.

Check your answers on p 164

13 At 0300 hours, 2 L of 0.9% sodium chloride is set up to be delivered through an infusion pump at 85 mL/hr. After 8 hours the prescribed rate is increased to 120 mL/hr. Calculate the finishing time.

14 A one litre IV flask of normal saline has been running at 90 mL/hr for 6 hours. A specialist then prescribes the rate to be increased so that the remaining solution will be infused in the next 4 hours. Calculate the new flow rate in mL/hr.

15 A post-operative patient is prescribed morphine 25 mg in 50 mL of normal saline via an infusion pump.

　a Calculate the concentration (mg/mL) of the morphine/saline solution.

　b How many milligrams of morphine will the patient receive hourly if the pump is set at 5 mL/hr?

　c At what rate (mL/hr) should the pump be set to deliver morphine at 3.5 mg/hr?

16 A post-operative patient is receiving a PCA infusion of fentanyl 250 micrograms in 25 mL of normal saline via a syringe pump. The PCA is set to give a bolus dose of 1 mL each time the button is pressed.

　a What is the concentration (microgram/mL) of the fentanyl/saline solution?

　b How much fentanyl is in each bolus dose?

　c If the patient has five bolus doses between 1400 hours and 1500 hours on a Sunday, how much fentanyl has the patient received in that hour?

17 One gram of dextrose provides 16 kJ of energy. How many kilojoules does a patient receive from an infusion of 1.5 L of 5% dextrose?

Check your answers on p 164

5 | Paediatric dosages

In this chapter dosages of medications for children will be considered. The exercises focus on the arithmetic of oral medications and injections *specifically for children*. Intravenous infusion calculations have been covered in Chapter 4.

The skills covered in this chapter will include medication calculations relating to both body weight and body surface area.

> Great care must be taken when administering medication to children. *The smallest error is potentially life-threatening*.

WHAT YOU NEED TO KNOW

Children grow at different rates.

There are wide variations in the actual weight of a child of a given age compared to the average weight for a child of that age. Consequently, dosages are usually calculated according to body weight. In more complex situations dosages are based on body surface area, for example in chemotherapy.

Body surface area can be determined using the body weight and height of a child. When dealing with an infant (a child aged less than 1 year), body weight and *length* are used.

Body surface area determines the loss of fluid from the body by evaporation. This fluid loss is critical in the case of some medications and this is when body surface area is used in a calculation, rather than weight.

The prescription should specify whether to use weight or body surface area.

> **Important**: If in **any** doubt about the answer to a calculation, then ask a supervisor to check your work.

Refer to prelim page ix for explanations of abbreviations.

CHAPTER CONTENTS

CALCULATING A SINGLE DOSE BASED ON BODY WEIGHT

Calculating the size of a single dose is based on the recommended dosage (in milligrams per kilogram per day) and a child's weight. The nurse is not usually required to do this calculation. However, it is important that you understand how a single dose prescription is determined.

Note: There is no particular formula required for these calculations.

Example A *A young girl is to be given amoxicillin. The recommended dosage is 30 mg/kg 12 hourly. The girl's weight is 18 kg. How much amoxicillin should she receive in each 12 hours?*

$$30 \text{ mg/kg} \times 18 \text{ kg} = 540 \text{ mg}$$

Example B *A child is prescribed erythromycin. The recommended dosage is 40 mg/kg/day, 4 doses daily. If the child's weight is 15 kg, calculate the size of a single dose.*

$$15 \text{ kg} \times 40 \text{ mg/kg/day} = 600 \text{ mg/day}$$

Then

$$600 \text{ mg} \div 4 \text{ doses} = 150 \text{ mg/dose}$$

Example C *A child is to be given ampicillin. The recommended dosage is 80 mg/kg/day, 4 doses per day. Calculate the size of a single dose if the child's weight is 27 kg.*

$$27 \text{ kg} \times 80 \text{ mg/kg/day} = 2160 \text{ mg/day}$$

Then

$$2160 \text{ mg} \div 4 \text{ doses} = 540 \text{ mg/dose}$$

Exercise 5A

Given each child's weight, calculate the amount of medication to be given 12 hourly.
1. Trimethoprim, 4 mg/kg, 12 hourly, weight 7 kg
2. Phenytoin, 3 mg/kg, 12 hourly, weight 33 kg
3. Spironolactone, 25 mg/kg, 12 hourly, weight 27 kg

Calculate the size of a single dose for a child weighing 12 kg.
4. Erythromycin, 40 mg/kg/day, 4 doses per day
5. Penicillin V, 50 mg/kg/day, 4 doses per day
6. Cefalexin, 30 mg/kg/day, 4 doses per day

Calculate the size of a single dose for a child weighing 20 kg.
7. Cloxacillin, 50 mg/kg/day, 4 doses per day
8. Chloramphenicol, 40 mg/kg/day, 4 doses per day
9. Amoxicillin, 45 mg/kg/day, 4 doses per day

Calculate the size of a single dose for a child weighing 36 kg.
10. Flucloxacillin, 100 mg/kg/day, 4 doses per day
11. Capreomycin sulphate, 20 mg/kg/day, 3 doses per day
12. Cephalothin, 60 mg/kg/day, 4 doses per day

Check your answers on p 165

ESTIMATING VOLUMES FOR INJECTION IN PAEDIATRIC PATIENTS

Example *A girl is to be given 150 micrograms of digoxin IV. Ampoules contain digoxin 0.5 mg in 2 mL. Is the volume to be drawn up for injection equal to 2 mL, less than 2 mL or more than 2 mL?*

Stock ampoule contains 0.5 mg of digoxin
0.5 mg = 500 micrograms
Volume of ampoule = 2 mL
150 micrograms (prescribed) is *less than* 500 microgram (stock)
Therefore, volume to be drawn up is *less than* 2 mL

Exercise 5B *Choose the correct answer to each problem. The answer will be equal to, less than, or more than the volume of the stock ampoule or vial.*

1   *Prescribed:* pethidine 30 mg
    Stock: pethidine 50 mg in 1 mL
    Is the volume to be drawn up equal to 1 mL, less than 1 mL or more than 1 mL?

2   *Prescribed:* capreomycin sulphate 200 mg
    Stock: capreomycin sulphate 1 g in 5 mL
    Is the volume to be drawn up equal to 5 mL, less than 5 mL or more than 5 mL?

3   *Prescribed:* gentamicin 25 mg
    Stock: gentamicin 20 mg/2 mL
    Is the volume to be drawn up equal to 2 mL, less than 2 mL or more than 2 mL?

4   *Prescribed:* naloxone 20 micrograms
    Stock: naloxone 0.02 mg/ mL
    Is the volume to be drawn up equal to 1 mL, less than 1 mL or more than 1 mL?

5   *Prescribed:* atropine 0.5 mg
    Stock: atropine 0.2 mg in 1 mL
    Is the volume to be drawn up equal to 1 mL, less than 1 mL or more than 1 mL?

6   *Prescribed:* flucloxacillin 350 milligrams
    Stock: flucloxacillin 1 g in 3 mL
    Is the volume to be drawn up equal to 3 mL, less than 3 mL or more than 3 mL?

Check your answers on p 165

CALCULATING VOLUMES FOR INJECTION IN PAEDIATRIC PATIENTS

Example A *A boy is prescribed pethidine 35 mg, IM at 0800 hours. Stock ampoules contain 50 mg in 1 mL. What volume must be drawn up for injection?*

$$\text{Volume required} = \frac{\text{Strength required}}{\text{Stock strength}} \times [\text{Volume of stock solution}]$$

The formula can be abbreviated to:

$$VR = \frac{SR}{SS} \times VS$$

$$= \frac{35\,mg}{50\,mg} \times 1\,mL$$

$$= \frac{35}{50}\,mL = \frac{7}{10}\,mL$$

$$= 0.7\,mL$$

Example B *A child is prescribed digoxin 40 micrograms, IV. Paediatric ampoules contain 50 micrograms/2 mL. Calculate the amount to be drawn up in a syringe.*

$$\text{Volume required} = \frac{\text{Strength required}}{\text{Stock strength}} \times [\text{Volume of stock solution}]$$

$$VR = \frac{SR}{SS} \times VS$$

$$= \frac{40\,micrograms}{50\,micrograms} \times 2\,mL$$

$$= \frac{40}{50} \times \frac{2}{1}\,mL$$

$$= \frac{80}{50}\,mL$$

$$= \frac{8}{5}\,mL$$

$$= 1.6\,mL$$

If you are having difficulty simplifying the fractions in these examples, then refer to Review exercises 1H and 1I in Chapter 1.

Exercise 5C *For each of these paediatric dosages calculate the volume to be drawn up in a syringe for injection.*

	Prescribed	Stock
1	Pethidine 20 mg	50 mg in 1 mL
2	Pethidine 10 mg	25 mg per mL
3	Metoclopramide 4 mg	10 mg in 2 mL
4	Atropine 0.3 mg	0.4 mg in 1 mL
5	Digoxin 125 micrograms	0.5 mg/2 mL
6	Digoxin 18 micrograms	50 micrograms in 2 mL
7	Capreomycin sulphate 200 mg	1 g in 2 mL
8	Capreomycin sulphate 150 mg	1 g in 5 mL
9	Cephalothin 120 mg	500 mg in 2 mL
10	Cephalothin 300 mg	500 mg in 2 mL
11	Flucloxacillin 400 mg	1 g in 3 mL
12	Flucloxacillin 100 mg	1 g in 3 mL
13	Phenobarbital 50 mg	200 mg/mL
14	Aminophylline 180 mg	250 mg in 10 mL
15	Morphine 6.5 mg	10 mg in 1 mL
16	Gentamicin 15 mg	20 mg/2 mL
17	Gentamicin 40 mg	60 mg/1.5 mL
18	Morphine 8 mg	10 mg/mL
19	Furosemide (frusemide) 4.5 mg	20 mg in 2 mL
20	Omnopon 16 mg	20 mg per mL
21	Naloxone 0.03 mg	0.02 mg/mL
22	Naloxone 0.05 mg	0.02 mg/mL

Always check that each answer makes sense.

Should the volume you calculated be equal to, or less than, or more than the volume of the stock ampoule?

Check your answers on p 165

CALCULATING PAEDIATRIC DOSAGES FOR ORAL MEDICATIONS IN LIQUID FORM

Children are frequently prescribed oral medication in liquid form. Liquid medication allows a greater range of specific dosages compared to solid form (tablets and capsules). This is especially relevant for children as there is a great range of weights for a child of a given age. Generally a child finds a liquid medication easier to take than a tablet or capsule. The liquid medication may be a syrup, an elixir, a solution or a suspension.

Important: Suspensions must be shaken thoroughly before measuring the volume.

Example A *A child is prescribed 80 mg of paracetamol elixir at 1000 hours. Stock on hand is 100 mg in 5 mL. Calculate the volume to be given.*

$$\text{Volume required} = \frac{\text{Strength required}}{\text{Stock strength}} \times [\text{Volume of stock solution}]$$

The formula can be abbreviated to:

$$VR = \frac{SR}{SS} \times VS$$

$$= \frac{80 \, mg}{100 \, mg} \times 5 \, mL$$

$$= \frac{80}{100} \times \frac{5}{1} \, mL$$

$$= \frac{4}{\cancel{5}} \times \frac{\cancel{5}}{1} \, mL \qquad [\text{The 5s cancel out}]$$

$$= 4 \, mL$$

Example B *A child is to be given 175 micrograms of digoxin, orally. Paediatric mixture contains 50 micrograms per mL. Calculate the required volume.*

$$\text{Volume required} = \frac{\text{Strength required}}{\text{Stock strength}} \times [\text{Volume of stock solution}]$$

The formula can be abbreviated to:

$$VR = \frac{SR}{SS} \times VS$$

$$= \frac{175 \, \text{micrograms}}{50 \, \text{micrograms}} \times 1 \, mL$$

$$= \frac{175}{50} \, mL$$

$$= \frac{35}{10} \, mL$$

$$= \frac{7}{2} \, mL$$

$$= 3.5 \, mL$$

Exercise 5D *Calculate the volume to be given orally for these paediatric dosages.*

	Prescribed	Stock
1	70 mg of paracetamol elixir	100 mg/5 mL
2	300 mg of paracetamol elixir	120 mg/5 mL
3	12.5 mg of promethazine elixir	5 mg/5 mL
4	70 mg of theophylline syrup	50 mg/5 mL
5	125 micrograms of digoxin elixir	50 micrograms/mL
6	24 mg of phenytoin suspension	30 mg/5 mL
7	200 mg of penicillin suspension	125 mg/5 mL
8	350 mg of penicillin suspension	125 mg/5 mL
9	60 mg of theophylline syrup	80 mg/15 mL
10	225 mg of amoxicillin syrup	1 g/10 mL
11	1.5 mg of clonazepam syrup	2.5 mg/mL
12	50 mg of amoxicillin syrup	1 g/10 mL
13	100 mg of flucloxacillin syrup	125 mg/5 mL
14	180 mg of flucloxacillin syrup	150 mg/5 mL

Check your answers on p 165

CALCULATING PAEDIATRIC DOSAGES INVOLVING POWDER-FORM MEDICATIONS FOR INJECTION

Some medications are supplied in vials containing the medication in powder form. The powder must be mixed with water-for-injection (WFI) before administration. When a known volume of WFI is mixed with the vial of powder, the resulting solution has a volume greater than the volume of the WFI. The concentration of the solution (mg/mL) depends upon the volume of WFI used. Some medication labels show the various amounts of WFI to be added to the vial to yield given concentrations of solutions.

VOLUME OF WATER-FOR-INJECTION AND CONCENTRATION OF A SOLUTION

Here is an example of a water-for-injection (WFI) table. The amoxicillin in the vial is in powder form.

Amoxicillin 500 mg IV vial

For concentration of:	100	125	200	250	mg/mL
Add:	4.6	3.6	2.1	1.6	mL of WFI

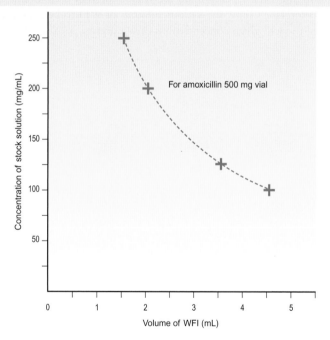

Figure 5.1 Showing relationship between concentration of a stock solution and volume of WFI.

The table and the graph show how the concentration of a stock solution depends on the volume of WFI mixed with the vial of powder. The bigger the volume of WFI, the lower the concentration of the stock solution.

Example *Stock vial: benzylpenicillin 600 mg*

For concentration of:	150	200	300	mg/mL
Add:	3.6	2.6	1.6	mL of WFI

A 12 kg child is prescribed 270 mg of benzylpenicillin, 8-hourly, IV. How much solution should be drawn up for injection if the concentration, after dilution with WFI, is each of the following:

a   150 mg/mL   b 200 mg/mL   c 300 mg/mL?

$$\text{Volume required} = \frac{\text{Strength required}}{\text{Stock strength}} \times [\text{Volume of stock solution}]$$

a   Volume required $= \dfrac{270 \text{ mg}}{150 \text{ mg}} \times 1 \text{ mL}$

$= \dfrac{9}{5} \text{ mL}$

$= 1.8 \text{ mL}$

$$5 \overline{)9.^40}$$
$$\underline{1.8}$$

b   Volume required $= \dfrac{270 \text{ mg}}{200 \text{ mg}} \times 1 \text{ mL}$

$= \dfrac{27}{20} \text{ mL}$

$= 1.35 \text{ mL}$

$= 1.4 \text{ mL}$ (correct to 1 d.p.)

$$10 \overline{)27.0}$$
$$2 \overline{)2.7^10}$$
$$\underline{1.35}$$

c   Volume required $= \dfrac{270 \text{ mg}}{300 \text{ mg}} \times 1 \text{ mL}$

$= \dfrac{9}{10} \text{ mL}$

$= 0.9 \text{ mL}$

Nursing Calculations

Exercise 5E *Give answers greater than 1 mL correct to one decimal place and answers less than 1 mL correct to two decimal places.*

1   An 8 kg child is prescribed 180 mg of benzylpenicillin, IV. How much solution should be drawn up for injection for the following concentrations after dilution with WFI (see benzylpenicillin table on page 123):
     a 150 mg/mL   b 200 mg/mL   c 300 mg/mL?

2   *Prescription:* amoxicillin 150 mg IV
     What volume of solution would need to be drawn up for injection for the following concentrations after dilution with WFI (see amoxicillin table on page 122):
     a 100 mg/mL   b 125 mg/mL   c 200 mg/mL   d 250 mg/mL?

3   *Label on vial:* Ampicillin 500 mg multiple-dose vial
     Reconstitution: Add 1.8 mL of WFI to yield 250 mg/mL
     What volume of the reconstituted mixture should be drawn up for injection if the prescription is for:
     a 100 mg   b 150 mg   c 200 mg of ampicillin?

4   *Label on vial*: Keflin 1 gram
     Reconstitution: Add 4 mL of WFI to yield 0.5 g/2.2 mL
     Calculate the volume of reconstituted mixture to be drawn up for injection if the prescription is for:
     a 200 mg   b 300 mg   c 350 mg of Keflin.

Check your answers on p 166

DETERMINING A CHILD'S BODY SURFACE AREA USING A NOMOGRAM

The dosages for the administration of medication to paediatric patients may be based on *body surface area*. Body surface area is a major factor in heat loss and moisture loss from the body. For most medications the weight of a child is used to calculate the dosage. However, when using certain medications (e.g. cytotoxic medication, which can have severe side effects), body surface area gives a more precise measurement than weight.

Figure 5.2 is a chart called a nomogram that relates a person's height (or length), weight and body surface area. Once the height (or length) and weight of a patient have been measured, then the body surface area can be determined using the nomogram.

BSA on the nomogram stands for *body surface area*.

Children of the same age have a wide range of heights (or lengths) and weights and, consequently, a wide range of body surface areas.

For instance, if a child has a height of 85 cm and a weight of 15 kg, then the child's body surface area is found by linking the height and weight measurements with a straight edge (e.g. a ruler): the area is 0.61 m^2.

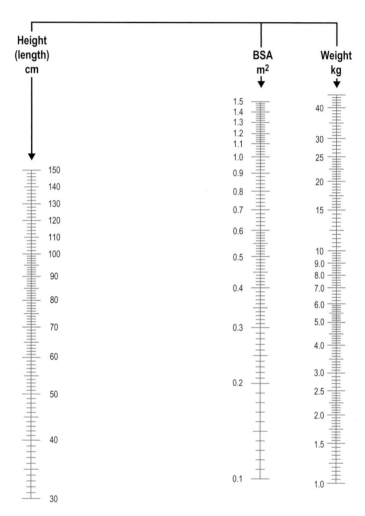

Figure 5.2 Nomogram for calculating body surface area (BSA). BSA is calculated by linking height (or length) and weight with a straight edge (use a ruler).

Example A *Using the nomogram in Figure 5.2, find the body surface area of an infant, aged 6 months, with a length of 65 cm and weight of 8.2 kg.*

On the nomogram, join length 66 cm and weight 8.2 kg with a straight edge (e.g. ruler). The straight edge then crosses the body surface area scale (marked BSA) at 0.40 m².

Example B *Using the nomogram in Figure 5.2, determine the body surface area of a boy of 2 years of age, height 87 cm, weight 13.5 kg.*

On the nomogram, join height 87 cm and weight 13.5 kg with a straight edge. The straight edge then crosses the body surface area scale at 0.58 m².

Nursing Calculations

Exercise 5F *The lengths (heights) and weights used below represent children from 3 months to 3 years of age. Use the nomogram in Figure 5.2 to find the body surface area of each child. Estimate answers to the nearest 0.01 m².*

Estimate answers to the nearest 0.01 m².

1   a   Length 65 cm, weight 6.4 kg
    b   Length 65 cm, weight 8.2 kg

2   a   Length 73 cm, weight 8.8 kg
    b   Length 73 cm, weight 10.5 kg

3   a   Length 85 cm, weight 11.0 kg
    b   Length 85 cm, weight 13.5 kg

4   a   Height 94 cm, weight 12.5 kg
    b   Height 94 cm, weight 15.5 kg

5   a   Weight 5.7 kg, length 57 cm
    b   Weight 5.7 kg, length 63 cm

6   a   Weight 9.4 kg, length 68 cm
    b   Weight 9.4 kg, length 74 cm

7   a   Weight 11.5 kg, length 78 cm
    b   Weight 11.5 kg, length 86 cm

8   a   Weight 14.0 kg, height 87 cm
    b   Weight 14.0 kg, height 97 cm

9   a   Length 67 cm, weight 10.0 kg
    b   Length 78 cm, weight 9.0 kg

10 a   Weight 13.0 kg, height 90 cm
    b   Weight 14.0 kg, height 81 cm

Check your answers on p 166

CALCULATING PAEDIATRIC DOSAGES BASED ON BODY SURFACE AREA

Example *A young patient with leukaemia is to be given his weekly injection of doxorubicin. The recommended dosage is 30 mg/m² and the boy's BSA has been determined at 0.48 m². Stock solution contains doxorubicin 10 mg/5 mL. Calculate the volume to be drawn up for injection.*

$$\text{Dose required (mg)} = \text{Body surface area (m}^2) \times \text{Recommended dosage (mg/m}^2)$$
$$= 0.48 \text{ m}^2 \times 30 \text{ mg/m}^2$$
$$= 14.40 \text{ mg}$$

$$\text{Volume required} = \frac{\text{Strength required}}{\text{Stock strength}} \times [\text{Volume of stock solution}]$$

$$VR = \frac{SR}{SS} \times VS$$

$$= \frac{14.4 \text{ mg}}{10 \text{ mg}} \times 5 \text{ mL}$$

$$= \frac{14.4}{10} \times \frac{5}{1} \text{ mL} \quad [\text{Divide the 5 and the 10 by 5}]$$

$$= \frac{14.4}{2} \text{ mL}$$

$$= 7.2 \text{ mL}$$

Exercise 5G

The aim of this exercise is to introduce the method of calculating medication doses based on body surface area. These doses are used in complex situations, such as the treatment of children with leukaemia, and are administered under very strict procedures and supervision.

Calculate the volume required in each case.

1   *Prescribed:* dactinomycin
    Recommended dosage: 1.5 mg/m^2
    Stock strength: 500 micrograms/mL
    Body surface area: 0.40 m^2

2   *Prescribed:* bleomycin
    Recommended dosage: 10 units/m^2
    Stock strength: 15 units/5 mL
    Body surface area: 0.54 m^2

3   *Prescribed:* cytarabine
    Recommended dosage: 120 mg/m^2
    Stock strength: 100 mg/5 mL
    Body surface area: 0.45 m^2

4   *Prescribed:* daunorubicin
    Recommended dosage: 30 mg/m^2
    Stock strength: 20 mg/5 mL
    Body surface area: 0.52 m^2

5   *Prescribed:* vincristine
    Recommended dosage: 1.5 mg/m^2
    Stock strength: 1 mg/mL
    Body surface area: 0.64 m^2

6   *Prescribed:* cyclophosphamide
    Recommended dosage: 1000 mg/m^2
    Stock strength: 1 g/50 mL
    Body surface area: 0.57 m^2

Check your answers on p 166

CHAPTER 5 REVISION

1   A child is prescribed cloxacillin. The recommended dosage is
    50 mg/kg/day, 4 doses daily. Calculate the size of a *single* dose if
    the child's weight is 22 kg.

2   A young boy weighing 19 kg is to be given cephalothin. The
    recommended dosage is 60 mg/kg/day, 4 doses daily. What should
    be the size of a *single* dose?

3   The recommended dosage for capreomycin sulphate is 20 mg/kg/
    day, 3 doses daily. Calculate the size of a *single* dose for a girl
    weighing 27 kg.

4   *Prescribed:* gentamicin 45 mg
    Stock: gentamicin 60 mg/1.5 mL
    Is the volume to be drawn up equal to 1.5 mL, less than 1.5 mL or
    more than 1.5 mL?

5   A girl is prescribed pethidine 15 mg. Stock ampoules on hand
    contain 50 mg in 2 mL. What volume must be withdrawn for
    injection?

6   A child is prescribed amoxicillin 320 mg. Stock contains 1 g in
    3 mL. What volume should be injected?

7   An injection of morphine 4 mg is prescribed. Calculate the amount
    to be drawn up if an ampoule contains 10 mg/1.5 mL.

8   A child is prescribed 180 mg of paracetamol. Stock elixir contains
    120 mg/5 mL. Calculate the volume to be given orally.

9   A boy is prescribed clonazepam 1.8 mg, orally. What volume of
    syrup should be administered if stock contains 2.5 mg/mL?

10 A young patient is prescribed penicillin 300 mg. The suspension on
    hand has a strength of 125 mg/5 mL. How much suspension should
    be given?

Check your answers on p 167

11 A girl is to receive amoxicillin 160 mg IV. What volume of solution should be drawn up for injection if the concentration, after dilution with WFI, is:

a 100 mg/mL   b 200 mg/mL   c 250 mg/mL?

12 A vial of ampicillin 500 mg is reconstituted with 1.8 mL of WFI to give a concentration of 250 mg/mL. Calculate the volume of this solution that should be drawn up for injection if the prescription is for:

a 75 mg   b 80 mg   c 175 mg   d 180 mg

Use the nomogram on page 126 *to work out the answers to questions 13–16.*

13 Find the body surface area of a girl of age 4 years, height 102 cm and weight 16.5 kg.

14 A boy of age 5 years has a height of 108 cm and weighs 18.5 kg. Find his body surface area.

15 A girl is 7 years of age. Her height is 120 cm and weight 20.5 kg. What is her body surface area?

16 A boy aged 8 weighs 24 kg and has a height of 124 cm. Determine his body surface area.

17 A boy is prescribed bleomycin. The recommended dosage is 10 units per m^2. Reconstituted stock has a strength of 15 units/5 mL. What volume should be injected if the boy has a BSA of 0.48 m^2?

18 A young patient is prescribed doxorubicin. The recommended dosage is 30 mg/m^2 and stock contains 50 mg/25 mL. Calculate the volume required if the patient's body surface area is 0.70 m^2.

Check your answers on p 167

Revision of nursing calculations | 6

The following three exercises revise the calculations covered in Chapters 2–5.

Revision exercise 6A

1   250 mg of soluble paracetamol is required. Stock on hand is 500 mg tablets. How many tablets should be given?

2   Warfarin tablets are available in strengths of 1 mg, 2 mg, 5 mg and 10 mg. Choose the best combination of whole tablets for each of the following dosages of warfarin: **a** 4 mg **b** 8 mg **c** 12 mg

3   A solution contains paracetamol 120 mg/5 mL. How many milligrams of paracetamol are in **a** 15 mL **b** 25 mL **c** 40 mL of the solution?

4   A patient is prescribed 360 mg of penicillin PO at 1400 hrs. The strength of the stock syrup is 125 mg per 5 mL. Calculate the volume required.

5   A patient is prescribed benzylpenicillin 1200 mg IV at 1230 hrs. Stock ampoules contain 1 g in 5 mL. Is the volume to be drawn up for injection equal to 5 mL, less than 5 mL or more than 5 mL?

6   Stock ampoules of erythromycin contain 300 mg/10 mL. Calculate the volume required for injection when a patient is prescribed erythromycin 135 mg IM.

7   400 mg of benzylpenicillin is to be given IV. On hand is benzylpenicillin 600 mg in 2 mL. What volume should be drawn up?

8   *Prescribed:* erythromycin 250 mg
    Stock: 300 mg in 10 mL
    Calculate the volume to be drawn up for injection.

Check your answers on p 168

9 A male patient is receiving one litre of 5% dextrose at a rate of 25 mL/hr. How much of the solution will he receive over **a** 3 hr **b** 5 hr **c** 12 hr?

10 A patient is to receive 200 mL of 0.9% sodium chloride IV. The infusion pump is set to deliver 120 mL/hr. How long will the infusion take?

11 One litre of Hartmann's solution is to be given over 12 hours. Calculate the required flow rate of a volumetric infusion pump. Give answer to the nearest whole number.

12 140 mL of fluid containing 600 mg of vancomycin is to be given over 50 minutes. Calculate the required pump setting in mL/hr.

13 700 mL of Hartmann's solution is to be given over 8 hours. The IV set delivers 20 drops/mL. What is the required drip rate?

14 A patient is to be given one unit of packed cells over 3 hours at 0330 hrs. Calculate the drip rate in drops/min if the unit of packed cells holds 250 mL and the giving set emits 20 drops per mL. Give the answer to the nearest whole number.

15 At 1100 hours on a Thursday, one litre of 4% dextrose and 0.18% sodium chloride is set up to run at 60 mL/hr. When will the flask finish?

16 At 0900 hrs on a Wednesday, one litre of 5% dextrose is set up to run over 9 hours. At what flow rate should the volumetric pump be set? Give answer to nearest whole number.

17 800 mL of fluid is to be given IV. The fluid is run at 70 mL/hr for the first 5 hours, then the rate is reduced to 60 mL/hr. Calculate the total time taken to give the 800 mL.

Check your answers on p 168

18 A patient is prescribed pethidine 400 mg in 500 mL of normal saline. The solution is to be infused via an infusion pump at between 10 and 40 mL/hr, depending on the nurse's assessment of the patient's pain.

   a Calculate the concentration of the pethidine in saline solution.

   b How many milligrams of pethidine will the patient receive hourly if the pump is run at 15 mL/hr?

   c At what rate should the pump be set to deliver 20 mg/hr? Give the answer to the nearest whole number.

19 One gram of dextrose provides 16 kJ of energy. How many kilojoules does a patient receive from an infusion of half a litre of 10% dextrose?

20 A child is prescribed penicillin V. The recommended dosage is 50 mg/kg/day, 4 doses daily. If the child's weight is 18 kg, calculate the size of a single dose.

21 *Prescribed:* digoxin 175 micrograms
Stock: digoxin 0.5 mg in 2 mL
Is the volume to be drawn up equal to 2 mL, less than 2 mL or more than 2 mL?

22 A girl is prescribed phenobarbitone 140 mg at 1430 hours. Stock ampoules contain 200 mg/mL. What volume must be withdrawn for injection?

23 A child is prescribed 175 mg of capreomycin sulphate by IM injection. A stock ampoule contains 1 g in 2 mL. What volume of stock should be drawn up in the syringe?

24 A young boy is to have 125 micrograms of digoxin, PO. Paediatric mixture has a strength of 50 micrograms per mL. Calculate the required volume.

25 A young patient is to be given benzylpenicillin 175 mg. What volume of solution should be drawn up for injection if the concentration, after dilution with water-for-injection, is a 300 mg/mL b 200 mg/mL c 150 mg/mL?

Check your answers on p 168

26 Using the nomogram on page 126, find the body surface area of a girl of age 9 months, length 68 cm and weight 9.2 kg.

27 A child is prescribed dactinomycin IV. The recommended dosage is 0.9 mg/m^2 and stock on hand has a strength of 500 micrograms/mL. Calculate the volume to be injected if the child's body surface area is 0.55 m^2.

Check your answers on p 168

Revision exercise 6B

1   How many 30 mg tablets of phenobarbitone should be given if phenobarbitone 15 mg is prescribed?

2   Thioridazine tablets are available in strengths of 10 mg, 25 mg, 50 mg and 100 mg. What combination of whole tablets should be used for dosages of **a** 60 mg **b** 85 mg **c** 110 mg?

3   A solution contains fluoxetine 20 mg/5 mL. How many milligrams of fluoxetine are in **a** 15 mL **b** 30 mL **c** 35 mL of the solution?

4   900 mg of benzylpenicillin is to be given orally at 1000 hrs. Stock mixture contains 250 mg/5 mL. Calculate the volume of mixture to be given.

5   Capreomycin sulphate 900 mg is prescribed. Stock ampoules contain 1 g in 3 mL. Is the volume required for injection equal to 3 mL, less than 3 mL or more than 3 mL?

6   An injection of digoxin 225 micrograms is prescribed. Stock on hand is digoxin 500 micrograms in 2 mL. What volume of stock should be given?

7   A patient is to receive a dose of gentamicin 140 mg IV. If stock ampoules contain 100 mg in 2 mL, calculate the volume to be drawn up for injection.

8   *Prescribed:* naloxone 0.25 mg
    Stock: 0.4 mg/mL
    How much stock solution should be drawn up for injection?

9   A young male patient is receiving 0.9% sodium chloride via IV infusion. The drip rate is adjusted to 20 mL/hr. How much solution will he receive over **a** 4 hr **b** $7\frac{1}{2}$ hr **c** $10\frac{1}{2}$ hr?

10 A patient is to receive one litre of normal saline IV. The infusion pump is set at 80 mL/hr. How long will the fluid last?

Check your answers on p 169

11 Over a period of 9 hours, a patient is to receive half a litre of 4% dextrose and $\frac{1}{5}$ normal saline via a volumetric infusion pump. At what flow rate should the pump be set? Give answer to nearest whole number.

12 150 mL of fluid containing 1.5 g of flucloxacillin is to be infused over 45 minutes at 1530 hours. Calculate the required pump setting in mL/hr.

13 A child is prescribed 120 mL of Hartmann's solution to be given over 5 hours. The microdrip delivers 60 drops/mL. Calculate the required drip rate in drops/min.

14 A unit of autologous blood is to be given to a patient over 4 hours. The unit of blood contains 480 mL and the giving set delivers 20 drops/mL. Calculate the drip rate in drops/min.

15 At 2200 hours on a Wednesday, 1 L of Hartmann's solution is set to run at 80 mL/hr. When will the infusion be finished?

16 A patient is prescribed 1.25 litres of 4% dextrose and 0.18% sodium chloride over 20 hours. Calculate the required flow rate setting for a volumetric infusion pump. Give answer to the nearest whole number.

17 A patient is to be given 1.2 litres of fluid IV. An infusion pump is set at a rate of 60 mL/hr. After 12 hours the rate is increased to 96 mL/hr. Calculate the total running time.

18 A post-operative patient is to receive a PCA infusion of fentanyl 350 micrograms in 35 mL of normal saline, via a syringe pump. The PCA is set to give a bolus dose of 1 mL each time the button is pressed.
   a What is the concentration of the fentanyl in saline solution?
   b How much fentanyl is in each bolus dose?
   c If the patient has four bolus doses between 1100 and 1200 hours on a Friday, how much fentanyl has the patient received in that hour?

Check your answers on p 169

19 One gram of dextrose provides 16 kJ of energy. A patient is given an infusion of 2 L of 4% dextrose and $\frac{1}{5}$ normal saline. How many kilojoules does this infusion provide?

20 A child is to be given capreomycin sulphate. The recommended dosage is 20 mg/kg/day, 3 doses per day. Calculate the size of a single dose if the child's weight is 24 kg.

21 *Prescribed:* pethidine 30 mg
   Stock: pethidine 25 mg in 1 mL
   Is the volume to be drawn up equal to 1 mL, less than 1 mL or more than 1 mL?

22 It is necessary to give an infant an injection of digoxin 35 micrograms. Paediatric ampoules contain 50 micrograms per 2 mL. Calculate the amount to be drawn up.

23 A boy is prescribed 120 mg of paracetamol elixir PO at 1700 hrs. Stock on hand has a strength of 100 mg/5 mL. What volume should be given?

24 A young girl is prescribed 700 mg of sulfadiazine, to be taken orally. The stock mixture contains 500 mg/5 mL. How much mixture should be given?

25 A vial of amoxicillin 500 mg is reconstituted with WFI to give a concentration of 200 mg/mL. Calculate the volume of this solution to be drawn up for injection if the prescription is for **a** 50 mg **b** 90 mg **c** 120 mg.

26 Using the nomogram on page 126, determine the body surface area of a boy 2 years of age, height 87 cm and weight 13.5 kg.

27 A young girl is to be given cytarabine IV. The recommended dosage is 150 mg/m^2. The girl's body surface area is determined as 0.60 m^2. Stock on hand has a strength of 500 mg/25 mL. What volume should be drawn up for injection?

Check your answers on p 169

Revision exercise 6C

1 How many 50 mg tablets of atenolol are needed for a dose of atenolol 125 mg?

2 Diazepam tablets are available in strengths of 2 mg, 5 mg and 10 mg. Choose the best combination of *whole* tablets for the following dosages: a 8 mg b 12 mg c 16 mg.

3 A solution contains chlorpromazine 25 mg/5 mL. How many milli-grams of chlorpromazine are in a 15 mL b 25 mL c 45 mL of the solution?

4 A patient is prescribed 175 mg of phenytoin. Stock suspension contains phenytoin 125 mg/5 mL. Calculate the volume required.
   [Note: Remember to shake the suspension before measuring the volume.]

5 A patient is to receive an injection of digoxin 350 micrograms. On hand are digoxin ampoules containing 500 micrograms in 2 mL. Is the volume required for injection equal to 2 mL, less than 2 mL or more than 2 mL?

6 Stock ampoules of pethidine contain 100 mg in 2 mL. If a patient is to receive 65 mg of pethidine by IM injection, calculate the volume of stock required.

7 A patient is to be given gentamicin 30 mg IM. Stock ampoules of gentamicin contain 80 mg/2 mL. Calculate the volume required for injection.

8 *Prescribed:* heparin 1250 units
   Stock: 1000 units per mL
   What volume of stock solution should be drawn up for injection?

9 A young woman is receiving Hartmann's solution intravenously at a rate of 120 mL/hr. How much solution will she receive over a 3 hr b 7 hr c 10 hr?

Check your answers on p 170

10 A male patient is to be given 600 mL of 0.9% sodium chloride IV. The drip rate is adjusted to deliver 25 mL/hr. What time will it take to administer the 600 mL?

11 One litre of normal saline is to be administered over $7\frac{1}{2}$ hours. Calculate the required flow rate of a volumetric infusion pump in mL/hr, to the nearest whole number.

12 70 mL of fluid containing 600 mg of penicillin has been added to a burette. The infusion is to be administered over 45 minutes. Calculate the required pump setting in mL/hr, to the nearest whole number.

13 An adult female is to be given half a litre of 0.9% sodium chloride over 6 hours. The administration set gives 20 drops/mL. Calculate the required drip rate in drops/min.

14 One unit of packed cells is to be run over $3\frac{1}{2}$ hours. The unit of packed cells contains 350 mL. If an IV set that emits 15 drops/mL is to be used, calculate the drip rate in drops per minute.

15 At 0530 hours Saturday an infusion pump is set to deliver 1.2 litres of fluid at a rate of 90 mL/hr. Calculate finishing time for the infusion.

16 A 1 litre IV flask of normal saline is to be infused over 11 hours. Calculate the required flow rate setting for a volumetric infusion pump. Give answer to the nearest whole number.

17 For 5 hours, a 1 litre IV flask has been running at 80 mL/hr. A specialist then orders the rate to be increased so that the remaining solution will be infused in the next 6 hours. Calculate the new flow rate in mL/hr.

18 An adult patient is prescribed morphine 45 mg in 500 mL of 0.9% sodium chloride at 10–40 mL/hr. A volumetric infusion pump is to be used to infuse the solution.
   a Calculate the concentration (mg/mL) of the morphine/saline solution.
   b How many milligrams of morphine will the patient receive hourly
   - if the pump is set at 25 mL/hr?
   c At what rate should the pump be set to deliver morphine 3 mg/hr? Give answer to the nearest whole number.

Check your answers on p 170

Nursing Calculations

19 One gram of glucose provides 16 kJ of energy. A patient is to receive an infusion of 750 mL of 5% glucose. How many kilojoules will the patient receive?

20 The recommended dosage for amoxicillin is 45mg/kg/day, 4 doses per day. Calculate the size of a single dose for a boy weighing 32 kg.

21 *Prescribed:* morphine 7.5 mg
   Stock: morphine 10 mg/mL
   Is the volume to be drawn up equal to 1 mL, less than 1 mL or more than 1 mL?

22 A girl is prescribed pethidine 45 mg, IM. Stock ampoules contain 50 mg in 1 mL. What volume must be withdrawn for injection?

23 A child is to be given 250 mg flucloxacillin IV. If stock ampoules contain 1 g in 3 mL, calculate the volume to be drawn up for injection.

24 A girl is prescribed 150 mg of amoxicillin syrup. Stock mixture contains 1 g/10 mL. How much syrup should be given?

25 *Label on vial:* cephalothin 1 gram
   Reconstitution: Add 4 mL of WFI to yield 0.5 g/2.2 mL
   Calculate the volume of reconstituted mixture to be drawn up for injection if the prescription is for **a** 150 mg **b** 250 mg **c** 450 mg of cephalothin.

26 Using the nomogram on page 126 determine the body surface area of an infant, aged 7 months, with a length of 69 cm and weight of 8.4 kg.

27 A young boy is prescribed daunorubicin. The recommended dose is 30 mg/m^2. Stock strength is 20 mg/5 mL. Calculate the volume to be drawn up for injection if the boy's body surface area is 0.56 m^2.

Check your answers on p 170

CHAPTER 1: A REVIEW OF RELEVANT CALCULATIONS

Diagnostic test

					Review exercise
1	a 830	b 8300	c 83 000		1A
2	a 0.258	b 2.58	c 25.8		1A
3	a 0.378	b 0.0378	c 0.00378		1B
4	a 56.9	b 5.69	c 0.569		1B
5	a 1000	b 1000	c 1000	d 1000	1C
6	a 830 g	b 6.4 kg			1C
7	a 780 mg	b 0.034 g			1C
8	a 86 micrograms	b 0.294 mg			1C
9	a 2400 mL	b 0.965 L			1C
10	a 70 mL	b 7 mL	c 0.07 L is larger		1D
11	a 45 mg	b 450 mg	c 0.45 g is heavier		1D
12	a 27	b 2.7	c 0.27	d 0.0027	1E
13	a 468	b 4.68	c 4.68	d 0.468	1E
14	2, 3, 4, 6 and 12 are factors				1F
15	2, 3, 6, 7 and 9 are factors				1F
16	a $\frac{2}{3}$	b $\frac{7}{9}$			1G
17	a $\frac{3}{40}$	b $\frac{7}{16}$			1G
18	a $\frac{4}{5}$	b $\frac{2}{3}$	c $\frac{3}{5}$		1H
19	a $\frac{7}{10}$	b $\frac{4}{5}$	c $\frac{2}{5}$		1H
20	a $\frac{13}{4}$	b $\frac{11}{2}$	c $\frac{25}{4}$		1I
21	a $\frac{35}{6}$	b $\frac{16}{5}$	c $\frac{12}{5}$		1I
22	a $\frac{2}{3}$	b $\frac{9}{10}$	c $\frac{400}{9}$	d $\frac{9}{5}$	1J
23	a 0.7	b 1.8	c 0.4		1K
24	a 0.37	b 2.63	c 0.52		1K

Review exercise 1A *Multiplication by 10, 100 and 1000*

1	6.8, 68, 680	9	0.147, 1.47, 14.7
2	9.75, 97.5, 975	10	0.06, 0.6, 6
3	37, 370, 3700	11	37.6, 376, 3760
4	56.2, 562, 5620	12	6.39, 63.9, 639
5	770, 7700, 77 000	13	0.75, 7.5, 75
6	8250, 82 500, 825 000	14	0.8, 8, 80
7	2, 20, 200	15	0.03, 0.3, 3
8	0.46, 4.6, 46	16	0.505, 5.05, 50.5

Review exercise 1B *Division by 10, 100 and 1000*

1	9.84, 0.984, 0.0984	9	6.8, 0.68, 0.068
2	0.591, 0.0591, 0.00591	10	0.229, 0.0229, 0.00229
3	0.26, 0.026, 0.0026	11	5.14, 0.514, 0.0514
4	30.7, 3.07, 0.307	12	91.6, 9.16, 0.916
5	8.2, 0.82, 0.082	13	6.72, 0.672, 0.0672
6	0.7, 0.07, 0.007	14	38.7, 3.87, 0.387
7	0.3, 0.03, 0.003	15	0.894, 0.0894, 0.00894
8	0.75, 0.075, 0.0075	16	0.0707, 0.00707, 0.000707

Review exercise 1C *Converting units*

Grams

1 5000	2 2400	3 750	4 1625

Kilograms

5 7	6 0.935	7 0.085	8 0.003

Milligrams

9 4000	10 8700	11 690	12 20
13 35	14 6	15 655	16 4280

Grams

17 6	18 7.25	19 0.865	20 0.095
21 0.07	22 0.002	23 0.005	24 0.125

Micrograms

25 195	26 600	27 750	28 75
29 80	30 1	31 625	32 98

Milligrams

33 0.825	34 0.75	35 0.065	36 0.095
37 0.01	38 0.005	39 0.2	40 0.03

Millilitres

41 2000	42 30000	43 1500	44 4500
45 1600	46 2240	47 800	48 750

Litres

49 4	50 10	51 0.625	52 0.35
53 0.095	54 0.06	55 0.005	56 0.002

Review exercise 1D *Comparing measurements*

1	a 100 mL	b	10 mL	c	0.1 L
2	a 3 mL	b	300 mL	c	0.3 L
3	a 50 mL	b	5 mL	c	0.05 L
4	a 47 mL	b	470 mL	c	0.47 L
5	a 400 mg	b	4 mg	c	0.4 g
6	a 60 mg	b	600 mg	c	0.6 g
7	a 70 mg	b	7 mg	c	0.07 g
8	a 630 mg	b	63 mg	c	0.63 g
9	a 2 micrograms	b	20 micrograms	c	0.02 mg
10	a 900 micrograms	b	90 micrograms	c	0.9 mg
11	a 1 microgram	b	100 micrograms	c	0.1 mg
12	a 580 micrograms	b	58 micrograms	c	0.58 mg
13	a 1500 g	b	1050 g	c	1.5 kg
14	a 2080 g	b	2800 g	c	2.8 kg
15	a 950 g	b	95 g	c	0.95 kg
16	a 3350 g	b	3500 g	c	3.5 kg

Review exercise 1E *Multiplication of decimals*

1   45, 4.5, 0.45, 0.45
2   14, 0.14, 0.014, 0.0014
3   12, 0.12, 0.12, 0.0012
4   36, 0.36, 0.0036, 0.0036
5   56, 5.6, 0.56, 0.0056
6   102, 10.2, 1.02, 0.102
7   152, 15.2, 0.152, 0.152
8   46, 0.46, 0.046, 0.0046
9   145, 1.45, 1.45, 1.45
10   93, 0.93, 0.0093, 0.093
11   333, 33.3, 0.333, 0.0333
12   287, 0.287, 0.0287, 2.87
13   192, 0.0192, 0.192, 0.0192
14   616, 6.16, 0.0616, 0.616
15   768, 0.768, 0.0768, 0.0768

Review exercise 1F *Factors*

1	2, 4, 5	11	4, 9, 12, 18
2	3, 4, 12	12	3, 5, 12, 15
3	3, 5, 15	13	3, 5, 9, 15
4	2, 8, 14	14	4, 8, 12, 16, 18, 24
5	3, 4, 12, 15, 20	15	5, 15, 25
6	3, 4, 6, 12, 18	16	3, 5, 11, 15
7	3, 5, 15, 25	17	5, 7
8	5, 17	18	4, 12, 15
9	3, 8, 12, 16, 24	19	4, 6, 8, 12, 16
10	5, 20, 25	20	6, 14, 15

Review exercise 1G *Simplifying fractions I*

Part i

1	$\frac{2}{3}$	6	$\frac{5}{7}$	11	$\frac{7}{8}$	16	$\frac{1}{3}$	21	$\frac{9}{14}$
2	$\frac{5}{7}$	7	$\frac{5}{6}$	12	$\frac{2}{3}$	17	$\frac{2}{3}$	22	$\frac{4}{5}$
3	$\frac{3}{8}$	8	$\frac{4}{5}$	13	$\frac{3}{7}$	18	$\frac{7}{8}$	23	$\frac{13}{16}$
4	$\frac{1}{2}$	9	$\frac{3}{7}$	14	$\frac{8}{9}$	19	$\frac{18}{25}$	24	$\frac{3}{10}$
5	$\frac{3}{4}$	10	$\frac{3}{10}$	15	$\frac{2}{5}$	20	$\frac{5}{11}$	25	$\frac{4}{9}$

Part ii

1	$\frac{1}{2}$	5	$\frac{1}{2}$	9	$\frac{2}{15}$	13	$\frac{5}{8}$	17	$\frac{7}{9}$
2	$\frac{3}{8}$	6	$\frac{5}{12}$	10	$\frac{8}{35}$	14	$\frac{3}{4}$	18	$\frac{3}{4}$
3	$\frac{3}{10}$	7	$\frac{5}{16}$	11	$\frac{3}{10}$	15	$\frac{11}{16}$	19	$\frac{17}{24}$
4	$\frac{1}{4}$	8	$\frac{1}{4}$	12	$\frac{4}{25}$	16	$\frac{4}{9}$	20	$\frac{13}{30}$

Nursing Calculations

Review exercise 1H *Simplifying fractions II*

1	$\dfrac{3}{5}$	7	$\dfrac{13}{15}$	13	$\dfrac{2}{3}$	19	$\dfrac{2}{3}$	25	$\dfrac{2}{3}$	31	$\dfrac{5}{6}$
2	$\dfrac{2}{3}$	8	$\dfrac{2}{3}$	14	$\dfrac{2}{5}$	20	$\dfrac{3}{4}$	26	$\dfrac{8}{15}$	32	$\dfrac{1}{6}$
3	$\dfrac{3}{4}$	9	$\dfrac{2}{5}$	15	$\dfrac{9}{10}$	21	$\dfrac{9}{10}$	27	$\dfrac{5}{6}$	33	$\dfrac{3}{20}$
4	$\dfrac{5}{12}$	10	$\dfrac{3}{4}$	16	$\dfrac{3}{5}$	22	$\dfrac{3}{4}$	28	$\dfrac{14}{25}$	34	$\dfrac{3}{8}$
5	$\dfrac{2}{3}$	11	$\dfrac{5}{8}$	17	$\dfrac{9}{10}$	23	$\dfrac{15}{16}$	29	$\dfrac{4}{5}$	35	$\dfrac{3}{10}$
6	$\dfrac{5}{6}$	12	$\dfrac{3}{8}$	18	$\dfrac{6}{25}$	24	$\dfrac{2}{5}$	30	$\dfrac{7}{10}$	36	$\dfrac{11}{16}$

Review exercise 1l *Simplifying fractions III*

1 a $\dfrac{3}{2}$ b $\dfrac{5}{2}$ c $\dfrac{15}{4}$ d $\dfrac{17}{4}$

2 a $\dfrac{25}{2}$ b $\dfrac{75}{4}$ c $\dfrac{75}{2}$ d $\dfrac{375}{4}$

3 a $\dfrac{25}{2}$ b $\dfrac{175}{6}$ c $\dfrac{125}{3}$ d $\dfrac{250}{3}$

4 a $\dfrac{5}{2}$ b $\dfrac{15}{2}$ c $\dfrac{19}{2}$ d $\dfrac{55}{4}$

5 a $\dfrac{7}{5}$ b $\dfrac{3}{2}$ c $\dfrac{12}{5}$ d $\dfrac{5}{2}$

6 a $\dfrac{4}{3}$ b $\dfrac{5}{2}$ c $\dfrac{25}{2}$ d $\dfrac{50}{3}$

7 a $\dfrac{5}{4}$ b $\dfrac{5}{2}$ c $\dfrac{55}{8}$ d $\dfrac{25}{2}$

8 a $\dfrac{3}{2}$ b $\dfrac{5}{3}$ c $\dfrac{5}{2}$ d $\dfrac{15}{4}$

9 a $\dfrac{8}{5}$ b $\dfrac{12}{5}$ c $\dfrac{32}{5}$ d $\dfrac{36}{5}$

10 a $\dfrac{6}{5}$ b $\dfrac{14}{5}$ c $\dfrac{22}{5}$ d $\dfrac{38}{5}$

11 a $\dfrac{6}{5}$ b $\dfrac{3}{2}$ c $\dfrac{8}{3}$ d $\dfrac{19}{3}$

12 a $\dfrac{16}{5}$ b $\dfrac{18}{5}$ c $\dfrac{24}{5}$ d $\dfrac{36}{5}$

Nursing Calculations

Review exercise 1J *Simplifying fractions IV*

1	$\dfrac{4}{5}$	9	$\dfrac{5}{2}$	17	$\dfrac{5}{4}$	25	$\dfrac{1}{2}$
2	$\dfrac{3}{4}$	10	$\dfrac{19}{8}$	18	$\dfrac{2}{3}$	26	$\dfrac{3}{4}$
3	$\dfrac{3}{2}$	11	80	19	7	27	9
4	$\dfrac{3}{7}$	12	$\dfrac{200}{3}$	20	$\dfrac{1}{2}$	28	120
5	2	13	200	21	$\dfrac{3}{2}$	29	$\dfrac{5}{8}$
6	$\dfrac{7}{10}$	14	$\dfrac{200}{9}$	22	$\dfrac{1}{3}$	30	$\dfrac{5}{2}$
7	$\dfrac{9}{4}$	15	$\dfrac{1000}{11}$	23	$\dfrac{3}{4}$	31	$\dfrac{3}{2}$
8	$\dfrac{11}{2}$	16	$\dfrac{9}{2}$	24	$\dfrac{400}{3}$	32	$\dfrac{200}{7}$

Review exercise 1K *Rounding off decimal numbers*

Part i

1	0.9	5	0.6	9	2.4	13	1.1
2	0.5	6	1.0	10	1.1	14	3.0
3	0.9	7	1.6	11	0.2	15	1.0
4	0.7	8	1.2	12	2.7	16	0.8

Part ii

1	0.33	5	0.14	9	2.71	13	0.63
2	1.67	6	0.13	10	1.29	14	0.78
3	0.88	7	0.92	11	0.64	15	2.43
4	0.83	8	1.57	12	0.22	16	1.86

Review exercise 1L *Fraction to a decimal I*

1	0.5	7	0.125	13	0.04	19	0.275
2	0.25	8	0.875	14	0.32	20	0.675
3	0.75	9	0.05	15	0.68	21	0.02
4	0.2	10	0.35	16	0.88	22	0.14
5	0.6	11	0.65	17	0.025	23	0.42
6	0.8	12	0.95	18	0.225	24	0.86

Review exercise 1M *Fraction to a decimal II*

Part i

1	0.3	3	0.3	5	0.2	7	0.5
2	0.8	4	0.7	6	0.3	8	0.9

Part ii

1	0.67	3	0.86	5	0.89	7	0.91
2	0.17	4	0.44	6	0.36	8	0.42

Review exercise 1N *Fraction to a decimal III*

Part i

1	$33.3 \Rightarrow 33$	5	$18.7 \Rightarrow 19$	9	$20.8 \Rightarrow 21$	13	$46.8 \Rightarrow 47$
2	$83.3 \Rightarrow 83$	6	$31.2 \Rightarrow 31$	10	$45.8 \Rightarrow 46$	14	$53.1 \Rightarrow 53$
3	$166.6 \Rightarrow 167$	7	$14.4 \Rightarrow 14$	11	$34.2 \Rightarrow 34$	15	$27.7 \Rightarrow 28$
4	$183.3 \Rightarrow 183$	8	$28.8 \Rightarrow 29$	12	$42.8 \Rightarrow 43$	16	$61.1 \Rightarrow 61$

Part ii

1	$1.66 \Rightarrow 1.7$	5	$2.85 \Rightarrow 2.9$	9	$3.12 \Rightarrow 3.1$	13	$2.22 \Rightarrow 2.2$
2	$3.33 \Rightarrow 3.3$	6	$3.57 \Rightarrow 3.6$	10	$4.37 \Rightarrow 4.4$	14	$5.55 \Rightarrow 5.6$
3	$5.83 \Rightarrow 5.8$	7	$7.14 \Rightarrow 7.1$	11	$6.87 \Rightarrow 6.9$	15	$7.77 \Rightarrow 7.8$
4	$4.16 \Rightarrow 4.2$	8	$9.28 \Rightarrow 9.3$	12	$5.62 \Rightarrow 5.6$	16	$9.44 \Rightarrow 9.4$

Nursing Calculations

Review exercise 10 *Mixed numbers and improper fractions*

Part i

1	$2\dfrac{1}{2}$	5	$4\dfrac{5}{6}$	9	$25\dfrac{1}{2}$	13	$15\dfrac{5}{6}$	17	$26\dfrac{3}{5}$
2	$3\dfrac{2}{3}$	6	$5\dfrac{1}{7}$	10	$21\dfrac{2}{3}$	14	$14\dfrac{3}{7}$	18	$23\dfrac{5}{6}$
3	$4\dfrac{1}{4}$	7	$4\dfrac{5}{8}$	11	$17\dfrac{3}{4}$	15	$14\dfrac{1}{8}$	19	$22\dfrac{3}{7}$
4	$4\dfrac{2}{5}$	8	$5\dfrac{4}{9}$	12	$17\dfrac{1}{5}$	16	$13\dfrac{8}{9}$	20	$18\dfrac{4}{9}$

Part ii

1	$\dfrac{3}{2}$	5	$\dfrac{7}{2}$	9	$\dfrac{67}{6}$	13	$\dfrac{45}{2}$	17	$\dfrac{185}{6}$
2	$\dfrac{4}{3}$	6	$\dfrac{14}{3}$	10	$\dfrac{93}{7}$	14	$\dfrac{74}{3}$	18	$\dfrac{228}{7}$
3	$\dfrac{7}{4}$	7	$\dfrac{25}{4}$	11	$\dfrac{133}{8}$	15	$\dfrac{111}{4}$	19	$\dfrac{283}{8}$
4	$\dfrac{13}{5}$	8	$\dfrac{49}{5}$	12	$\dfrac{155}{9}$	16	$\dfrac{146}{5}$	20	$\dfrac{347}{9}$

Review exercise 1P *Multiplication of fractions*

1	$\dfrac{1}{5}$	7	$\dfrac{3}{5}$	13	$\dfrac{11}{42}$	19	$\dfrac{9}{10}$	25	$\dfrac{7}{15}$
2	$\dfrac{5}{24}$	8	$\dfrac{9}{20}$	14	$\dfrac{3}{140}$	20	$\dfrac{9}{32}$	26	$\dfrac{7}{16}$
3	$\dfrac{5}{9}$	9	$\dfrac{5}{6}$	15	$\dfrac{20}{21}$	21	1	27	$\dfrac{4}{27}$
4	$\dfrac{1}{6}$	10	$\dfrac{3}{20}$	16	$\dfrac{12}{35}$	22	$\dfrac{1}{135}$	28	$\dfrac{3}{16}$
5	$1\dfrac{2}{3}$	11	$\dfrac{4}{9}$	17	$\dfrac{5}{28}$	23	$\dfrac{7}{18}$	29	$\dfrac{2}{15}$
6	$\dfrac{3}{50}$	12	$\dfrac{1}{18}$	18	$\dfrac{1}{16}$	24	$\dfrac{5}{27}$	30	$\dfrac{1}{5}$

Review exercise 1Q *Multiplication of a fraction by a whole number*

Part i

1	$\dfrac{15}{4} = 3\dfrac{3}{4}$	4	$\dfrac{20}{3} = 6\dfrac{2}{3}$	7	$\dfrac{9}{2} = 4\dfrac{1}{2}$	10	$\dfrac{10}{3} = 3\dfrac{1}{3}$
2	$\dfrac{6}{5} = 1\dfrac{1}{5}$	5	6	8	$\dfrac{15}{8} = 1\dfrac{7}{8}$	11	$\dfrac{10}{3} = 3\dfrac{1}{3}$
3	4	6	$\dfrac{6}{7}$	9	4	12	$\dfrac{3}{5}$

Part ii

1	3.5	4	0.7	7	3.6	10	2.8
2	1.2	5	2.5	8	3.75	11	9
3	0.6	6	1.8	9	1.6	12	4.4

Review exercise 1R *24-hour time*

Part i

All answers are in hours.

1	0910	4	1105	7	1255	10	1735
2	2040	5	0400	8	1315	11	0745
3	0230	6	1525	9	0620	12	2250

Part ii

1	7:35 pm	4	2:00 am	7	9:25 pm	10	5:10 am
2	10:30 pm	5	1:05 pm	8	6:40 am	11	12:20 pm
3	1:05 am	6	5:45 pm	9	11:15 pm	12	2:50 pm

Part iii

All answers are in hours.

1	1745 Monday	5	0525 Monday
2	0530 Friday	6	1840 Wednesday
3	2015 Saturday	7	0020 Saturday
4	0400 Wednesday	8	1910 Thursday

CHAPTER 2: DOSAGES OF ORAL MEDICATIONS

Exercise 2A

1	2	3	$1\frac{1}{2}$	5	$1\frac{1}{2}$	7	$1\frac{1}{2}$	9	$2\frac{1}{2}$
2	$\frac{1}{2}$	4	2	6	$\frac{1}{2}$	8	$\frac{1}{2}$	10	$\frac{1}{2}$

Exercise 2B

1 a 2 mg + 2 mg (2 tablets)
   b 5 mg + 2 mg + 2 mg (3 tablets)
   c 10 mg + 2 mg (2 tablets)
   d 10 mg + 5 mg (2 tablets)

2 a 5 mg + 2 mg (2 tablets)
   b 5 mg + 2 mg + 2 mg (3 tablets)
   c 10 mg + 5 mg (2 tablets)
   d 10 mg + 10 mg (2 tablets)

3 a 120 mg + 80 mg (2 tablets); or 160 mg + 40 mg (2 tablets)
   b 120 mg + 120 mg (2 tablets); or 160 mg + 80 mg (2 tablets)
   c 160 mg + 120 mg (2 tablets)
   d 160 mg + 160 mg (2 tablets)

4 a 5 mg + 1 mg (2 tablets)
   b 5 mg + 2 mg + 1 mg (3 tablets)
   c 5 mg + 2 mg + 2 mg (3 tablets)
   d 5 mg + 5 mg + 1 mg (3 tablets)

5 a 40 mg + 20 mg (2 tablets)
   b 80 mg + 20 mg (2 tablets)
   c 80 mg + 80 mg + 40 mg (3 tablets)
   d 500 mg + 40 mg + 20 mg (3 tablets)

6 a 25 mg + 10 mg (2 tablets)
   b 50 mg + 10 mg (2 tablets)
   c 50 mg + 25 mg (2 tablets)
   d 100 mg + 10 mg + 10 mg (3 tablets)

Exercise 2C *All answers are in milligrams (mg).*

1 a 20	b 30	c 50
2 a 6	b 10	c 14
3 a 80	b 200	c 400
4 a 500	b 750	c 1000
5 a 40	b 100	c 160
6 a 500	b 1000	c 1500
7 a 50	b 150	c 250
8 a 750	b 1250	c 1750

Exercise 2D *All volumes are in millilitres (mL).*

1 20	4 7.5	7 7.5	10 24
2 4	5 6	8 20	11 32
3 2.5	6 25	9 7	

Exercise 2E

1 2 tablets	3 a (i) 10 mg (ii) 20 mg b 4 mL
2 2 tablets	4 a (i) 25 mg (ii) 50 mg b 8 mL

Chapter 2 Revision

If you make an error in answering any of the questions in the revision exercises, then refer back to the worked Examples in the corresponding exercises and also to the relevant Review exercises, given in brackets after each answer.

1 2 *[2A: 1I]*

2 $\frac{1}{2}$ *[2A : 1J]*

3 $1\frac{1}{2}$ *[2A : 1I]*

4 a 2 mg + 1 mg (2 tablets)

 b 5 mg + 2 mg (2 tablets)

 c 10 mg + 2 mg + 1 mg (3 tablets)

 d 10 mg + 5 mg + 1 mg (3 tablets) *[2B]*

5 Shaken thoroughly

6 a 50 mg

 b 100 mg

 c 250 mg *[2C: 1A]*

7 a 750 mg

 b 1250 mg

 c 1750 mg *[2C]*

8 15 mL *[2D: 1I, 1P, 1Q]*

9 25 mL *[2D: 1I, 1P, 1Q]*

10 16 mL *[2D: 1I, 1P, 1Q]*

11 15 mL *[2D: 1I, 1Q]*

12 2.5 mL *[2D: 1I, 1N]*

CHAPTER 3: DOSAGES OF MEDICATIONS FOR INJECTION

Exercise 3A

1	less than 1 mL	5	equal to 10 mL
2	more than 2 mL	6	less than 2 mL
3	less than 5 mL	7	more than 1 mL
4	more than 2 mL ·	8	more than 2 mL

Exercise 3B *All answers are in millilitres (mL). Volumes more than 1 mL are given to one decimal place; volumes less than 1 mL are given to two decimal places.*

1	0.80	3	0.90	5	1.3	7	1.5
2	1.4	4	2.5	6	1.7	8	3.0

Exercise 3C *All answers are in millilitres (mL). Volumes more than 1 mL are given to one decimal place; volumes less than 1 mL are given to two decimal places.*

1	5.0	4	4.0	7	1.3
2	3.2	5	0.80	8	1.6
3	0.50	6	0.20	9	0.55

Exercise 3D *All answers are in millilitres (mL). Volumes more than 1 mL are given to one decimal place; volumes less than 1 mL are given to two decimal places.*

1	1.2	4	1.6	7	0.60
2	1.5	5	4.0	8	0.60
3	2.5	6	1.5	9	$3.75 \Rightarrow 3.8$

Exercise 3E *All answers are in millilitres (mL).*

1	6.7	4	0.67	7	1.4
2	1.3	5	0.88	8	1.8
3	0.83	6	0.43	9	1.3

Exercise 3F *All answers are in millilitres (mL).*

1	0.80	5	0.35	9	3.0	13	1.8	17	1.3
2	0.28	6	1.6	10	2.5	14	3.8	18	0.75
3	12.5	7	1.2	11	4.0	15	0.75	19	6.0
4	0.60	8	0.80	12	2.4	16	3.8	20	1.3

Exercise 3G *All answers are in millilitres (mL).*

1	0.80	2	6.0	3	0.50	4	3.5

Exercise 3H

1 a $\frac{1}{100}$ mL = 0.01 mL   b A 0.20 mL   B 0.38 mL   C 0.73 mL
D 0.55 mL

2 a $\frac{1}{10}$ mL = 0.1 mL   b A 1.2 mL   B 2.15 mL   C 2.6 mL

3 a $\frac{1}{5}$ mL = 0.2 mL   b A 2.2 mL   B 4.5 mL   C 3.9 mL

4 a $\frac{1}{5}$ mL = 0.2 mL   b A 6.0 mL   B 3.4 mL   C 7.5 mL

5 a 2 units   b A 40 units   B 4 units   C 75 units   D 65 units

6 a 1 unit   b A 30 units   B 42 units   C 25 units   D 17 units

7 a $\frac{1}{2}$ unit = 0.5 unit   b A 40 units   B 36 units   C 27.5 units
D 32.5 units

Nursing Calculations

Chapter 3 Revision

If you make an error in answering any of the questions in the revision exercises, then refer back to the worked Examples in the corresponding exercises and also to the relevant Review exercises, given in brackets after each answer.

All volumes are in millilitres (mL). Volumes more than 1 mL are given to one decimal place; volumes less than 1 mL are given to two decimal places.

1 less than 1 mL *[3A]*
2 1.4 *[3B, 3C, 3D: 1B, 1H, 1P, 1Q]*
3 2.4 *[3B, 3C, 3D: 1G, 1H, 1N, IP, 1Q]*
4 7.5 *[3B, 3C, 3D: 1I, 1L, 1P, 1Q]*
5 1.1 *[3B, 3C, 3D: 1I, 1L, 1P, 1Q]*
6 1.5 *[3B, 3C, 3D: 1G, 1H, 1P, 1Q]*
7 9.0 *[3B, 3C, 3D: 1C, 1H, 1P, 1Q]*
8 0.90 *[3B, 3C, 3D: 1J, 1L, 1P, 1Q]*
9 6.33 $\Rightarrow$ 6.3 *[3E, 3F: 1H, 1K, 1M, 1P, 1Q]*
10 0.666 $\Rightarrow$ 0.67 *[3E, 3F: 1G, 1K, 1M]*

CHAPTER 4: INTRAVENOUS INFUSION

Exercise 4A

1	a 84 mL	b 336 mL	c 504 mL
2	a 375 mL	b 625 mL	c 1500 mL
3	a 90 mL	b 150 mL	c 720 mL
4	20 hours		

5 $12\frac{1}{2}$ hours $= 12$ hr 30 min

6 $6\frac{2}{3}$ hours $= 6$ hr 40 min

7 $\frac{2}{3}$ hr $= 40$ min

Exercise 4B *All answers are in mL/hr.*

1	125	6	$62.5 \Rightarrow 63$
2	$41.6 \Rightarrow 42$	7	$62.5 \Rightarrow 63$
3	$71.4 \Rightarrow 71$	8	$41.6 \Rightarrow 42$
4	$133.3 \Rightarrow 133$	9	$55.5 \Rightarrow 56$
5	$166.6 \Rightarrow 167$	10	$83.3 \Rightarrow 83$

Exercise 4C *All answers are in mL/hr.*

1	120	6	$106.6 \Rightarrow 107$
2	144	7	$112.5 \Rightarrow 113$
3	200	8	168
4	100	9	160
5	$102.8 \Rightarrow 103$	10	200

Exercise 4D *All answers are in drops/min.*

1	50	7	50
2	25	8	120
3	20.8 $\Rightarrow$ 21	9	40
4	13.8 $\Rightarrow$ 14	10	24
5	27.7 $\Rightarrow$ 28	11	80
6	33.3 $\Rightarrow$ 33	12	22.2 $\Rightarrow$ 22

Exercise 4E *All answers are in drops/min.*

1	20.8 $\Rightarrow$ 21	5	29.1 $\Rightarrow$ 29
2	41.6 $\Rightarrow$ 42	6	40
3	41.6 $\Rightarrow$ 42	7	34.2 $\Rightarrow$ 34
4	50	8	35

Exercise 4F

1	1530 hours Tuesday	5	2400 hours Monday (or 0000 hours Tuesday)
2	0100 hours Monday		
3	2130 hours Friday	6	0600 hours Sunday
4	0345 hours Friday	7	0030 hours Thursday

Exercise 4G

1 1800 mL or 1.8 L

2 Running time = $13\frac{1}{3}$ hr = 13 hr 20 min
   Finishing time = 0800 hr + 13 hr 20 min = 2120 hours

3 Running time = 20 hr
   Finishing time = 2100 hr Monday + 20 hr 00 min = 1700 hours Tuesday

4 6 hr + 7 hr = 13 hours

5 Total running time = 5 hr + $2\frac{1}{2}$ hr = $7\frac{1}{2}$hr = 7 hr 30 min
   Finishing time = 0800 hr + 7 hr 30 min = 1530 hours

6 Total running time = 10 hr + 8 hr = 18 hr
   Finishing time = 0430 hr + 18 hr 00 min = 2230 hours

7 110 mL/hr

8 55 mL/hr

Exercise 4H

1 a 0.7 mg/mL
   b i 7 mg   ii 10.5 mg   iii 17.5 mg   iv 28 mg
   c i 12.8 $\Rightarrow$ 13 mL/hr   ii 17.1 $\Rightarrow$ 17 mL/hr
      iii 28.5 $\Rightarrow$ 29 mL/hr   iv 35.7 $\Rightarrow$ 36 mL/hr

2 a 0.1 mg/mL
   b i 1 mg   ii 1.5 mg   iii 2 mg   iv 4 mg
   c i 15 mL/hr   ii 25 mL/hr   iii 30 mL/hr   iv 35 mL/hr

3 a 10 micrograms/mL   b 10 micrograms   c 60 micrograms

Exercise 4I *All answers are in kilojoules.*

1 800
2 2000
3 1600
4 2000

5 0 (no carbohydrate)
6 480
7 0 (no carbohydrate)
8 400

Chapter 4 Revision

If you make an error in answering any of the questions in the revision exercises, then refer back to the worked Examples in the corresponding exercises and also to the relevant Review exercises, given in brackets after each answer.

1   a 110 mL   b 275 mL   c 605 mL   *[4A]*

2   $8\frac{1}{3}$ hr = 8 hr 20 min   *[4A: 1C, 1I, 1O]*

3   75 mL/hr   *[4B: 1C, 1I]*

4   90.9 ⇒ 91 mL/hr   *[4B: 1C, 1I, 1K, 1N]*

5   133.3 ⇒ 133 mL/hr   *[4C: 1I, 1K, 1N, 1P]*

6   50 drops/min   *[4D: 1I, 1P]*

7   27.7 ⇒ 28 drops/min   *[4E: 1G, 1K, 1N, 1P]*

8   50 drops/min   *[4D: 1C, 1G, 1I, 1P]*

9   20.8 ⇒ 21 drops/min   *[4D: 1C, 1G, 1I, 1K, 1N, 1P]*

10 1620 mL or 1.62 L   *[4G]*

11 Running time = $12\frac{1}{2}$ hr = 12 hr 30 min

    Finishing time = 0700 hr + 12 hr 30 min = 1930 hours
    [4G: 1C, 1I, 1O, 1R]

12 6 hr + 11 hr = 17 hr   *[4G: 1C, 1I]*

13 Total running time = 8 hr + 11 hr = 19 hr
    Finishing time = 0300 hr + 19 hr 00 min = 2200 hours
    [4G: 1C, 1I, 1R]

14 115 mL/hr   *[4G: 1C, 1I, 1N]*

15 a 0.5 mg/mL   b 2.5 mg/hr   c 7 mL/hr   *[4H: 1B, 1E, 1G, 1J]*

16 a 10 micrograms/mL   b 10 micrograms   c 50 micrograms
    [4H: 1E, 1I]

17 1200 kJ   *[4I: 1C, 1H]*

CHAPTER 5: PAEDIATRIC DOSAGES

Exercise 5A *All answers are in milligrams (mg).*

1	28	4	120	7	250	10	900
2	99	5	150	8	200	11	240
3	675	6	90	9	225	12	540

Exercise 5B

1	less than 1 mL	3	more than 2 mL	5	more than 1 mL
2	less than 5 mL	4	equal to 1 mL	6	less than 3 mL

Exercise 5C *All answers are in millilitres (mL). Volumes more than 1 mL are given to one decimal place; volumes less than 1 mL are given to two decimal places.*

1	0.40	7	0.40	13	0.25	19	0.45
2	0.40	8	0.75	14	7.2	20	0.80
3	0.80	9	0.48	15	0.65	21	1.5
4	0.75	10	1.2	16	1.5	22	2.5
5	0.50	11	1.2	17	1.0		
6	0.72	12	0.30	18	0.80		

Exercise 5D *All answers are in millilitres (mL). Volumes more than 1 mL are given to one decimal place; volumes less than 1 mL are given to two decimal places.*

1	3.5	5	2.5	9	11.25 ⇒ 11.3	13	4.0
2	12.5	6	4.0	10	2.25 ⇒ 2.3	14	6.0
3	12.5	7	8.0	11	0.60		
4	7.0	8	14.0	12	0.50		

Nursing Calculations

Exercise 5E *All answers are in millilitres (mL).*

1	a	1.2	b	0.90	c	0.60	
2	a	1.5	b	1.2	c	0.75	d 0.60
3	a	0.40	b	0.60	c	0.80	
4	a	0.88	b	1.32 ⇒ 1.3	c	1.54 ⇒ 1.5	

Exercise 5F *All answers give body surface area (BSA) in m².*

1	a 0.35		5	a 0.31		9	a 0.45
	b 0.40			b 0.32			b 0.45
2	a 0.43		6	a 0.43		10	a 0.57
	b 0.48			b 0.45			b 0.57
3	a 0.51		7	a 0.51			
	b 0.57			b 0.53			
4	a 0.57		8	a 0.59			
	b 0.64			b 0.61			

Exercise 5G *All answers are in millilitres (mL).*

1	1.2	3	2.7	5	0.96
2	1.8	4	3.9	6	28.5

Chapter 5 Revision

If you make an error in answering any of the questions in the revision exercises, then refer back to the worked Examples in the corresponding exercises and also to the relevant Review exercises, given in brackets after each answer.

1   275 mg   *[5A]*
2   285 mg   *[5A]*
3   180 mg   *[5A]*
4   less than 1.5 mL   *[5B]*
5   0.60 mL   *[5C: 1G, 1L, 1P, 1Q]*
6   0.96 mL   *[5C: 1B, 1C, 1H, 1L, 1Q]*
7   0.60 mL   *[5C: 1E, 1G, 1L]*
8   7.5 mL   *[5D: 1I, 1N, 1P, 1Q]*
9   0.72 mL   *[5D: 1J, 1L]*
10   12.0 mL   *[5D: 1I, 1P, 1Q]*
11   a 1.6 mL   b 0.80 mL   c 0.64 mL   *[5E: 1H, 1I, 1L]*
12   a 0.30 mL   b 0.32 mL   c 0.70 mL   d 0.72 mL   *[5E: 1G, 1L]*
13   0.68 m²   *[5F]*
14   0.74 m²   *[5F]*
15   0.82 m²   *[5F]*
16   0.90 m²   *[5F]*
17   1.6 mL   *[5G: 1B, 1E, 1J, 1N, 1P]*
18   10.5 mL   *[5G: 1B, 1E, 1J, 1N, 1P]*

CHAPTER 6: REVISION OF NURSING CALCULATIONS

Note: If you make an error in answering any of the questions in these revision exercises, then refer back to the corresponding exercises in Chapters 2–5, provided in brackets after each answer below.

Revision exercise 6A

1 $\frac{1}{2}$ tablet *[2A]*

2 a 2 mg + 2 mg (2 tablets) b 5 mg + 2 mg + 1 mg (3 tablets)
   c 10 mg + 2 mg (2 tablets) *[2B]*

3 a 360 mg b 600 mg c 960 mg *[2C]*

4 14.4 mL *[2D]*

5 more than 5 mL *[3A]*

6 4.5 mL *[3B]*

7 1.33 $\Rightarrow$ 1.3 mL *[3C]*

8 8.33 $\Rightarrow$ 8.3 mL *[3E]*

9 a 75 mL b 125 mL c 300 mL *[4A]*

10 1 hr 40 min *[4A]*

11 83.3 $\Rightarrow$ 83 mL/hr *[4B]*

12 168 mL/hr *[4C]*

13 29.1 $\Rightarrow$ 29 drops/min *[4D]*

14 27.7 $\Rightarrow$ 28 drops/min *[4E]*

15 0340 hr Friday *[4G]*

16 111.1 $\Rightarrow$ 111 mL/hr *[4G]*

17 5 hr + 7$\frac{1}{2}$ hr = 12$\frac{1}{2}$ hr = 12 hr 30 min *[4G]*

18 a 0.8 mg/mL b 12.0 mg/hr c 25 mL/hr *[4H]*

19 800 kJ *[4I]*

20 225 mg/dose *[5A]*

21 less than 2 mL *[5B]*

22 0.70 mL *[5C]*

23 0.35 mL *[5D]*

24 2.5 mL *[5D]*

25 a 0.583 $\Rightarrow$ 0.58 mL b 0.875 $\Rightarrow$ 0.88 mL c 1.16 $\Rightarrow$ 1.2 mL *[5E]*

26 0.43 m^2 *[5F]*

27 0.99 mL *[5G]*

Revision exercise 6B

1   $\frac{1}{2}$ tablet   *[2A]*

2   **a** 50 mg + 10 mg (2 tablets)   **b** 50 mg + 25 mg + 10 mg (3 tablets)
   c 100 mg + 10 mg (2 tablets)   *[2B]*

3   **a** 60 mg   **b** 120 mg   **c** 140 mg   *[2C]*

4   18.0 mL   *[2D]*

5   less than 3 mL   *[3A]*

6   0.90 mL   *[3B]*

7   2.8 mL   *[3C]*

8   $0.625 \Rightarrow 0.63$ mL   *[3E]*

9   **a** 80 mL   **b** 150 mL   **c** 210 mL   *[4A]*

10   $12\frac{1}{2}$ hours = 12 hr 30 min   *[4A]*

11   $55.5 \Rightarrow 56$ mL/hr   *[4B]*

12   200 mL/hr   *[4C]*

13   24 drops/min   *[4D]*

14   40 drops/min   *[4E]*

15   Running time = 12 hr 30 min
   Finishing time = 1030 hours Thursday   *[4G]*

16   $62.5 \Rightarrow 63$ mL/hr   *[4G]*

17   12 hr + 5 hr = 17 hr   *[4G]*

18   **a** 10 micrograms/mL   **b** 10 micrograms/dose
   c 40 micrograms   *[4H]*

19   1280 kJ   *[4I]*

20   160 mg/dose   *[5A]*

21   more than 1 mL   *[5B]*

22   1.4 mL   *[5C]*

23   6.0 mL   *[5C]*

24   7.0 mL   *[5D]*

25   **a** 0.25 mL   **b** 0.45 mL   **c** 0.60 mL   *[5E]*

26   0.57m^2 *[5F]*

27   4.5 mL   *[5G]*

Revision exercise 6C

1 $2\frac{1}{2}$ tablets *[2A]*
2 a 2 mg + 2 mg + 2 mg + 2 mg (4 tablets) b 10 mg + 2 mg (2 tablets)
   c 10 mg + 2 mg + 2 mg + 2 mg (4 tablets) *[2B]*
3 a 75 mg b 125 mg c 225 mg *[2C]*
4 7.0 mL *[2D]*
5 less than 2 mL *[3A]*
6 1.3 mL *[3B]*
7 0.75 mL *[3C]*
8 1.25 $\Rightarrow$ 1.3 mL *[3E]*
9 a 360 mL b 840 mL c 1200 mL (or 1.2 L) *[4A]*
10 24 hr *[4A]*
11 133.3 $\Rightarrow$ 133 mL/hr *[4B]*
12 93.3 $\Rightarrow$ 93 mL/hr *[4C]*
13 27.7 $\Rightarrow$ 28 drops/min *[4D]*
14 25 drops/min *[4E]*
15 1850 hours Saturday *[4G]*
16 90.9 $\Rightarrow$ 91 mL/hr *[4G]*
17 100 mL/hr *[4G]*
18 a 0.09 mg/mL b 2.25 mg/hr c 33.3 $\Rightarrow$ 33 mL/hr *[4H]*
19 600 kJ *[4I]*
20 360 mg/dose *[5A]*
21 less than 1.5 mL *[5B]*
22 0.90 mL *[5C]*
23 0.75 mL *[5C]*
24 1.5 mL *[5D]*
25 a 0.66 mL b 1.1 mL c 1.98 $\Rightarrow$ 2.0 mL *[5E]*
26 0.41 m^2 *[5F]*
27 4.2 mL *[5G]*

Index

Page numbers followed by '*f*' indicate figures, and '*b*' indicate boxes.

Index

Index